DATE DUE

The Organ
Donor Experience

The Organ Donor Experience

Good Samaritans and the Meaning of Altruism

Katrina A. Bramstedt
and Rena Down

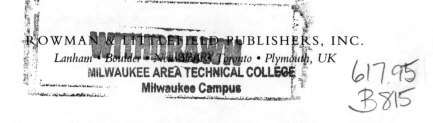

ROWMAN & LITTLEFIELD PUBLISHERS, INC.
Lanham • Boulder • New York • Toronto • Plymouth, UK

Published by Rowman & Littlefield Publishers, Inc.
A wholly owned subsidiary of The Rowman & Littlefield Publishing Group, Inc.
4501 Forbes Boulevard, Suite 200, Lanham, Maryland 20706
http://www.rowmanlittlefield.com
Estover Road, Plymouth PL6 7PY, United Kingdom

British Library Cataloguing in Publication Information Available

Library of Congress Cataloging-in-Publication Data

Bramstedt, Katrina.
    The organ donor experience : good samaritans and the meaning of altruism / Katrina A.
Bramstedt and Rena Down.
        p. cm.
    Summary: "Organ donors are, by definition, altruists, and their act is even more
generous when they remain anonymous. But altruism doesn't tell the whole story. There
are myriad motivations, some subconscious, some conscious, that compel people to
donate a part of themselves to someone they don't know. The Organ Donor Experience
uncovers the desires, personalities and motivations of Good Samaritan organ donors and
reveals much about the process of donating an organ to a needy recipient"— Provided by
publisher.
    Includes bibliographical references and index.
    ISBN 978-1-4422-1115-5 (hardback) — ISBN 978-1-4422-1117-9 (electronic)
    1. Organ donors. 2. Organ donors—Psychology. 3. Generosity. 4. Donation of
organs, tissues, etc. I. Title.
    RD129.5.B73 2011
    617.9'54—dc23   2011016618

♾™ The paper used in this publication meets the minimum requirements of
American National Standard for Information Sciences—Permanence of Paper
for Printed Library Materials, ANSI/NISO Z39.48-1992.

Printed in the United States of America

Contents

Foreword

$\mathcal{I}$ am delighted that the authors took the time to create such an informative and compelling book from the inspirational acts of the superheroes that we commonly refer to as Good Samaritan donors. If you are in doubt that there is good in this world, you need to read this book. You will be inspired.

A few words about my own transplant experience. When my youngest daughter was ten years old, her kidneys failed. When we learned that she would never recover her kidney function, it was clear that a living donor kidney transplant would give her the best outcome. I attempted to donate my kidney and proceeded through the evaluation process only to learn, thirty-six hours prior to surgery, that I failed the final cross-match test and would not be able to donate because my daughter would reject my kidney. I was devastated.

Our daughter finally received a kidney transplant after a difficult and extensive donor search. Fifteen donors were tested—one was compatible and could donate—my twenty-three-year-old nephew. He is our superhero and exemplifies those who walk among us and bring light to this world.

Collectively, Good Samaritan donors have saved the lives of over 200 people through donor chains organized by the National Kidney Registry over the past two years alone. I am honored to know many of the superheroes who fill the pages of this book. I continue to be awed by their selfless generosity and am amazed by the increasing number of Good Samaritan donors who are coming forward to give the gift of life to total strangers.

Read this book and be inspired!

Garet Hil
Founder and President
National Kidney Registry

Acknowledgments

This book would not have been possible were it not for the generosity of each Good Samaritan organ donor. Not only did they change the lives of their organ recipients, but they changed our lives as well. We remain forever amazed at their service to humanity and thank them for allowing us to explore their personal domains. We also express deep gratitude to the several transcriptionists who volunteered their time to work on this project, transcribing dozens of hours of interviews from audiocassette tapes to readable documents. Rena Down thanks her angel, Arlene Arthur, for her gift. We dedicate this book to all those who give the gift of life through organ donation.

Thank you.

Introduction

$\mathscr{I}$f you tell someone that you have donated an organ to a stranger (or that you want to), the reaction is likely to be one of astonishment and disbelief. *Why would anyone do that? Who are these Good Samaritans so committed to helping others—strangers—that they would undergo surgery, discomfort and disruption of their lives?* Our book explores these questions and more.

For the donor, altruism should be the primary motivation. Sometimes, the foundation is religious or spiritual—donors feeling a divine guidance to donate. For those who have a previous history of blood donation, they see their organ gift not as a sacrifice but as the next step in the helping process. But there are usually unconscious reasons as well for performing this great act of kindness. Our book gives twenty-two Good Samaritan organ donors (kidney, liver lobe, and lung lobe) the opportunity to tell their stories as they understand them. They are interviewed, and their transcripts and questionnaires are analyzed to discover the psychological and motivational underpinnings behind their extraordinary gift.

Although our sample is small, we've discovered some commonality among these donors. Most are younger or middle children, many profess religious beliefs that relate to their values, and nearly all are volunteers in their community. Many have served in the military or a parent did. Several work in the health care field or had the desire to do so as a child. While some of these traits are common to many people, few become living organ donors.

Dialysis centers are filled with patients who are in need of new kidneys. Some find themselves without a living donor because they have a limited circle of friends and family, and even when there is a willing volunteer, often the person is not an immunological match or medical issues eliminate the opportunity (e.g., high blood pressure or obesity). Others are sometimes

1

promised kidneys by friends or family only to be told that, for some reason, the individuals decided against it. The effect on the intended recipient can be traumatic. Hopes are raised and then dashed because the potential donor was either coerced by family members to donate or ambivalent. They mean well. They want to help. They go through the tests, but they back out. Why? Fear? Perhaps because they have no underlying "need" to donate. Though the procedure is always entirely voluntary, with a Good Samaritan, we suspect the likelihood of backing out is diminished because he or she often feels an innate drive to give.

In coming years, the need for organs will be even greater than it is now. The aging population and the epidemic of obesity almost ensure a rise in kidney failure. As of December 2010, more than 110,000 people were on a waiting list needing transplants in the United States.[1] About 28,000 transplants occur yearly, most of them via deceased donor organs.[2] A small percentage, about 6,200, received organs from living donors, most of them family members.[3] Of these living donors, about one hundred are "Good Samaritans."[4]

So what is a patient to do? Their options are limited. For those in kidney failure, they can remain on dialysis and hope to be transplanted before they die, but for those needing liver tissue, there is no bridge to save them while they wait. Some patients opt to leave the United States and go to a Third World country where poor-quality organs are regularly available for purchase (from the poor and others who cannot give informed consent to "donate"). Another option is to hope that they receive a living organ donation from a Good Samaritan before it's too late.

I (Rena Down) received my kidney from an anonymous donor. I was grateful and wanted to be able to give my donor something equally precious. Money, except for her out-of-pocket expenses, was out of the question—the sale of organs is illegal in the United States, as it is in most countries. I asked my donor why she felt the need to donate. She said, "Because I could."[5] I accepted that answer, although I felt that it was not the *only* truth. I was sure there had to be a reason she needed to donate beyond her ability to do so.

As a playwright and screenwriter, I know that a character's actions are the heart and spine of the story. And while nonfiction deals with facts, fiction frequently tells the truth by exploring the thoughts and feelings of characters and interpreting them in a way that nonfiction is unable to do. Our book marries the two forms. In order to get at the heart of the unconscious motivation of Good Samaritan organ donors, Dr. Bramstedt and I interviewed twenty-two of them and listened closely to what was being said and questioned their replies until they, themselves, understood why they felt the need to donate. By having donors tell their stories, they construct narratives that explain a lot about their motivations. What they say, what they don't say, what they imply, and what they want us to know about them enlightens us about their actions.

The subject of donors' motivations' interested me as material for a theater piece, but I wasn't sure know how best to approach the subject. Then, two years after my transplant, I read an article about a clinical ethicist, Dr. Katrina Bramstedt, at the time working at the California Pacific Medical Center in San Francisco, who did extensive interviews with prospective organ donors to determine whether they were suitable candidates.[6] I contacted her because I had begun to wonder if some of the interviews could be made into a theater piece—documentary theater, a form with which I'm familiar. Over lunch, as we talked about donors and their motivations, both of us began to realize that that this was a book that had to be written since the subject of Good Samaritan motivations had never been thoroughly explored. When I asked if the exploration of motivation would discourage potential donors, she said, "The ones who are unsuitable will be discouraged. The others will be interested to discover things about themselves and will proceed because, at heart, they are true altruists."[7]

Dr. Bramstedt had worked in the field of medical and transplant ethics for five years at the Cleveland Clinic before moving to the Bay Area of northern California. Prior to that, she spent two years as a fellow at the University of California, Los Angeles. She has written on the subject of donation and transplantation and lectures extensively. I, a professional writer, bring the seasoned ability to mold raw material into dramatic narratives and to shed light on the motivations of characters' actions. And, more important, I am able to draw on my own experience of dialysis and transplantation, the latter being the transforming experience of my life. Dr. Bramstedt and I are the perfect combination of experience and knowledge. As for the voices of the organ donors, they are the most critical part of this undertaking.

It seems that the act of Good Samaritan organ donation is extremely generous, in part because these donors don't choose their recipients, and, generally, they have no desire to even meet them. Deconstructing altruism in this situation is an enlightening and heartwarming experience. In our book, we discover the desires, personalities, and motivations of Good Samaritan organ donors. A sampling of these donor interviews are condensed into profiles.

RENA'S STORY

In February 2003, I lost the use of my kidneys. I told very few people about this catastrophe. I had worked in television for eighteen years and was fairly well known, and I was familiar enough with Hollywood and its culture to know that it was imperative that no one find out I was sick. While everyone in the media business voices sympathy to people with incurable diseases, business is business, and working in television is for the young and healthy, *not* the older and sick.

I was hospitalized in New York for six weeks and then was put on dialysis. After three years on dialysis, three hours a day, three days a week, a catheter in my chest, watching my blood circulate through a clear plastic tube as my body was being cleansed of "impurities," I realized I would be tied to a machine for the rest of my life if I didn't do something about it. Each dialysis session rendered me exhausted and unable to do anything but go to bed. I became seriously depressed and cut off contact with all but my closest friends. At the dialysis center, one could hear the same story coming from people younger than me who had been on dialysis for much longer, and I chided myself for complaining. My depression deepened, and I went into therapy. My therapist, recommended by a friend, was herself a transplant recipient. I realized that I had to become proactive and thus became determined to get a transplant.

At that time, the waiting list time for a deceased donor kidney in New York was between seven and ten years. My close family tried to help, but my daughter was a different blood type, one sister had hypertension, and the other was simply afraid. I was out of options from my family, so when a young friend offered her kidney, I was moved and grateful. I couldn't believe my good luck. I flew her to New York from San Francisco where she went through grueling tests for a week, met with social workers and psychiatrists, and was pronounced an excellent candidate. But after months of waiting for her to decide on a date for the transplant, she simply stopped communicating. No reason was given. Phone calls and emails were not returned, and I never heard from her again.

There comes a point of desperation when you'll do anything to find a donor. A friend, Paul, had received a kidney transplant in Peru and was back at work in three weeks. I phoned him. He told me about the operation and the excellent care he received afterward. He said the hospital was cleaner than any he had seen in the United States, and he gave me the name of the surgeon and suggested I call him.

My Spanish is not the best, but I managed to make an appointment to meet with the Peruvian surgeon. I arranged for dialysis at a clinic and flew to Lima. The hospital was as Paul had described it, and the dialysis center was far cleaner and more efficient than mine in New York. The doctors I met with could not have been nicer. The surgeon told me that he had performed more than three hundred transplants. In addition, there was no waiting list, which I found hard to believe. "Where do these donors come from?" I asked. "Religious people who want to do something for humanity," he told me.[8] I accepted this explanation because I wanted to.

I went to the dialysis center in Lima three times a week, and just before my last session, I noticed, for the first time, a bulletin board with notices such as "Woman, 25 years old, Type B Negative Offers Kidney" and "Man, 40 years of age, Type O Positive, Willing to Donate." Now, I became suspicious. *Were these people being paid?* "Of course they are," a nurse told me. "I thought they were religious people?" I said. "Some are. Most of them just need the money," she answered.[9]

Disheartened, I returned home to New York. Shortly thereafter, I received a phone call from Andrea, a woman with whom my friend Carol had worked. She told me that she was aware that I needed a kidney and that she might have a donor for me. It took a moment for this concept to register and for me to catch my breath. Then my left brain took over, and I became suspicious. *Was she kidding?* No, she was quite serious. In fact, she had the names of several people who were willing to donate. *How could this be?*

Andrea's brother needed a kidney. He was thirty-eight years old, the father of two small children. To help him, Andrea went on Craigslist,[10] a free advertising service on the Internet, and posted her brother's story. She received four hundred responses. Most of the responses were bogus, but a few were real possibilities. Andrea was featured on the front page of the *New York Daily News* since this was the first time someone actually admitted to having found a kidney on Craigslist. She particularly liked one woman, Arlene, who her brother had decided was too old to donate to him. *Did I want to talk to her?*

Instead of calling her immediately, I waited until I had relocated for the summer to San Francisco. Then I waited some more. I was frightened. I couldn't take another disappointment, and this all sounded too good to be true. Finally, I called Arlene, and she sounded lovely. She lived in southern California, and I invited her to come to San Francisco to meet me.

We could not be less alike. Arlene is a tall, blond athlete, and I am a short city type whose idea of athletics is running to Starbucks for another latte. She was divorced, as was I, and she has six children; I have one. She was a southerner from a military family; I'm a New Yorker from an eastern family—no member of which had ever voted Republican. However, she was willing to give me her kidney, and she was my angel.

I asked Arlene several times why she was doing this. "Because I can,"[11] was one answer. "I like to help people,"[12] was another. "I've donated blood. I am registered to donate marrow. Kidney donation is the logical next step."[13] Arlene wanted to be a nurse when she was young, but she married the first time at seventeen and became a mother at eighteen, which ended her health care dream. But those answers, while true, were not enough for me. There had to be another reason. It would be several years until I would gain further insight into her motivation.

We went through the donation and transplant operations at the University of California, San Francisco, and recovered together with the help of my sister, Shelly. Then Arlene returned home. We kept in touch, and she came to visit before I left California for New York. She stayed for several days. We toured the city, went hiking (her idea—not mine), and had several dinners at home. One night we began drinking a little too early, and by the time dinner was over, we were "relaxed." I had stopped asking her why she became a donor, but that night she offered some information about her life that she had neglected to tell me before.

Her father had killed himself when she was five years old. Her husband became an alcoholic and killed himself after she left him. One brother died in a biking accident, and another brother, a Vietnam vet, was homeless. (The year after the transplant, he was murdered during a drug deal.) She remarried. Her second husband brought three children to the marriage, and she decided to have two more of her own. Now she had six children to care for. Her husband left her soon after her last child was born, leaving his own three children behind. She eventually adopted them, and they are all devoted to her.

She had suffered so much loss in her life that I wondered if she donated her kidney out of some kind of guilt for having survived or because the losses made her feel that whatever she could do to save a life, she would do. She is a natural caretaker and cannot do enough to help people. But she is not a martyr. She loves her children and loves her life. Arlene sails, is active in a motorcycle club, and takes care of her twelve grandchildren whenever she can. But the need to donate blood, bone marrow, platelets, and a kidney comes from another place.

I tell you this because people like Arlene who donate organs to strangers while asking for nothing in return are, without question, altruists, but donation can also have side effects, and maybe it gives donors something they need, such as self-esteem, the admiration or approval of others, atonement for a misdeed, a new start in life, or the sense of honoring a personal or universal moral duty. I wondered about the motivations of other donors. *Were they making amends or looking for admiration? Were there other reasons for their actions? Did they, like Arlene, have particular life experiences that led them to do something as dramatic as donating a vital part of their body?* While I was pondering these questions and wondering how best to uncover the answers, I contacted the ethicist, Dr. Bramstedt, and we decided to collaborate on this book.

KATRINA'S STORY

My mother loves to retell the story of my taking my dolls and teddy bears with me to restaurants but never leaving behind my essential thermometer (hinged under an arm) so that I could take their temperature throughout the meal and keep my eye on their health all through the dinner hour.

I started out as a premed student and found my way into the field of medical device engineering, specifically cardiac implants. I became an expert at determining the root cause of why a particular device, returned by a surgeon, had failed on use. Years of investigating returned products led me down new paths of clinical intellectual curiosity, yet my mind kept returning to thoughts of the bioethics coursework I had taken as an undergraduate. Perhaps it was the lack of black-and-white answers that keep my brain churning over complex medical dilemmas, paired with my personality—I am a tenacious problem solver. I enrolled in a master's degree bioethics program, graduated, and moved on to a PhD and fellowship, which led me directly to the field of transplant ethics. Working as a hospital ethicist, my medical device knowledge was very helpful and allowed me to build relationships with many surgeons. It is within these relationships that the doctors found that we shared some common experiences and vocabulary, and they trusted me to help them.

At the time of my arrival into bioethics (1996), left-ventricular assist implants were emerging on the scene and presented complex ethical dilemmas never imagined. These are large metal devices that attach to a patient's heart through the chest cavity and function as a unique heart pump so that a sick heart can rest. Patients either wait for a new heart or use these devices as a permanent implant. Basically, the devices are a form of artificial life support. I was primed and ready to take on the ethical challenges and began proactively working with cardiac and transplant teams. From there, my work expanded to all solid organ transplant teams, even if a medical device was not involved. Teams found my knowledge and bedside skills extremely helpful.

In my role assessing potential living donors, I aim to be their advocate, looking after their safety and welfare. Sometimes, their personal situations cloud their objectivity, and they cannot give true informed consent. Sometimes, it is painfully clear that their motivation is not altruism. Sometimes, they look to ethicists to provide them with a way out, an excuse, because they don't want to donate at all but feel internal or external pressure to do so. As an ethicist, I do many things, including educating and resolving conflict. I seek to ensure that donations are without coercion and that they are informed, with an underpinning of altruism. Our book looks especially at the latter item. *What motivates a healthy person to have a vital organ removed from his or her body and given to a stranger? Who are these donors?* Our book presents both conceptual information about ethics and altruism as well as the personal stories of donors. Their motivations are often a complex weave of themes not easily categorized into tidy classification schemes. We attempted to blend the interviews with discussions of distinct ethical constructs and insert distinct story chapters alongside chapters with congruent themes; however, we make the stipulation that there are occasions where some stories are so multifaceted that there were multiple placement options. For clarification purposes, we don't want to give the impression that any one donor fits rigidly into only one topical theme in terms of their motivation for donation. Read on and step into the world of Good Samaritan organ donation.

Dr. Katrina Bramstedt

I

ETHICS AND ALTRUISM

• 1 •

Ethics, Values, Motivations

EXPLORING ALTRUISM

$\mathcal{D}$onation testimonies are often emotional and inspirational, but those features alone don't make a behavior "ethical." It is not enough that Good Samaritan organ donation be a safe and beneficent practice; it must also be ethically appropriate. Specifically, the *motives* of potential donors must be examined during their assessment process because there is the stipulation that organ donation, "the gift of life," is just that—a gift. This stipulation is based on the concept of altruism and originates from many sources, including the United Network for Organ Sharing and the American Society of Transplantation. This is further enunciated by regulations that forbid organ selling in the United States[1] and most other countries. Altruism is not only a concept but also the premise of organ donation. Further, it seems its most vivid form is evidenced in the act of Good Samaritan donation.

Altruism, defined as the "disinterested and selfless concern for the well-being of others," is derived from the Italian *altrui*, "somebody else."[2] What sets Good Samaritan donation apart from other forms of living organ donation is the fact that the recipient is an unknown individual—not a friend, relative, business partner, colleague, or associate. The concern and expressed behavior (donation) benefit someone with whom there is no emotional or genetic attachment. Further, both the concern and the expressed behavior are at extreme levels. The concern is so extreme that it moves the individual to undergo a personally unnecessary surgical procedure that is lifesaving for an unknown person.

Historically, the concept of being a Good Samaritan dates back to biblical times.[3] A Jewish traveler was beaten, robbed, and left nearly dead on a road. First a priest and then a Levite came by, but neither provided help. A Samaritan came by and gave aid, including cleaning and binding his wounds, taking him to shelter, and paying for his accommodation. Samaritans and Jews generally despised each other because of complex religious differences, and their leaders taught that it was wrong to have any contact with each other. Because these two groups were not to associate, the story of the Good Samaritan is a profound example of one party reaching out to another in an act of selflessness. Circling back to the original roadside injury response, the term "Good Samaritan" continues to be a widely used phrase in the health care setting, most prominently in organ donation, as well as the naming of twenty-three U.S. hospitals. Journalists even use the term when reporting on stories of individuals coming to the aid of stranded or injured travelers, as do the legislatures that draft laws to protect these first responders.

THEORIES OF ALTRUISM

Use of the term "altruism" began in the 1800s when it was coined by the French philosopher and sociologist August Comte. To this day, there are numerous theories as to the origins of altruistic behavior. Some pose that if there is any benefit at all to the person providing the help, then the helping act is not *really* altruistic. Some pose that altruism has genetic tendencies. Because it is impossible to capture and explain all these theories, we have selected a few of the most prominent for exploration. In a subsequent chapter, we also put forth our own theory of altruism.

Some believe that altruistic motivations arise from an altruistic personality and that people who have this personality are more inclined to behave altruistically than those who do not have this personality. For these people, on their palate of possible ways to respond to a situation, there are more altruistic options available to them compared to people who don't have an altruistic personality. They see ways to help and are willing to make choices that put their altruistic values into action. *How is it that these people have an altruistic personality?* Social psychologists think their experiences early in life are contributing factors. According to sociologists Samuel and Pearl Oliner, an altruistic personality is a "relatively ensuring predisposition to act selflessly on behalf of others."[4]

Some believe that there are universal ethical principles that spawn altruistic motivations. They believe that these ethical principles apply to everyone across all races, religions, political affiliations, genders, and creeds. This philosophical theory argues that a personal commitment to the universal ethical principles moves people to "do the right thing."[5] Another theory of altruism argues that some people set within themselves a *personal* code of conduct and beliefs according to which they act. This has been referred to as "internalized personal values."[6] Altruistic motivations arising from these personal internalized values can move the individual to act altruistically either as a form of "doing the right thing" or out of being concerned about the welfare of another person, depending on the nature of the personal belief system. Thus, the internalized personal values approach to altruism allows for a broad range of triggers for helping behavior. It potentially expands far beyond *just* "doing the right thing."

Philosopher Shaun Nichols has contrived a theory of altruism called the Concern Mechanism.[7] This theory has three elements: distressful input, change in feeling or emotion, and the altruistic act. As an example, a man sees a building on fire and hears screams coming from the second floor. The flames, smoke, heat, and screams cause him to feel urgent paternal rescue and nurturing emotions, and he runs into the building, up the stairs, and grabs a small child who is floundering in a dark hallway. *Was his behavior the "right thing to do"?* Yes, but it was more than that. The origin of the behavior was a motivation that had a caring component. Embedded in the nurturing and rescuing emotions was a caring component that was aligned with the child's welfare. He recognized suffering and responded with a behavior that provided aid.

Altruism is thought to be related to the ethics of care (which is related to virtue ethics). Ethics of care is a philosophical approach often seen in the caring professions, such as medicine and nursing; thus, it is no surprise that some of the Good Samaritan donors we interviewed were currently employed in a caring profession or that, as a child, that type of employment was their goal. Within the ethics-of-care approach to decision making, the caring components of a situation are morally important and can be in tension with formal rules and policies. For an individual who lives by the ethics of care approach, tuning in to what other people are feeling and needing is morally critical. Rules and policies can complicate the plans of people whose platform is caring. It is no wonder that several of the Good Samaritan donors we interviewed were perplexed at why transplant centers viewed their intentions as "too good to be true" and "overcomplicated" the donor candidate evaluation process. For these donors, it seemed that people who didn't understand their altruistic ways threw numerous roadblocks in their path (e.g., multiple psychiatric assessments and waiting periods). As Ken, a Good Samaritan liver donor, told us, "There are some people who just like to do good things and it's just that simple."[8]

ALTRUISM: BLACK, WHITE, OR GRAY?

For some, altruism can mean only one thing: *all* the benefits must go to the person getting the help. There is no gray zone that allows the giver to get any benefits, for this is seen as a contaminant to the altruistic motivation. Once altruism is contaminated, it is no longer altruism; rather, there is egoism at work. *But does it have to be this way? Might there be indirect consequences to the giver that are benefits but that were not the original goal? Do these indirect consequences really harm or negate the altruistic motive? Can altruism and indirect positive consequences for the giver exist in philosophical and ethical harmony?*

The expert on this topic is social psychologist C. Daniel Batson, and he has spent his life studying altruism, empathy, and prosocial behavior (e.g., providing comfort; sharing information, food, or other objects; and helping others achieve their goals). Dr. Batson makes numerous arguments supporting the fact that there can be multiple positive goals of a person's behavior. For example, if a person rendering aid to the needy gets some benefit along the way, this could be just an unintended consequence. It does not mean the motivation was not altruistic. His theory, the empathy-altruism hypothesis, makes room for the giver to also receive benefits in an indirect way.[9] Consider this example: I am a pilot flying an airplane with four other people on board when I notice that both engines are on fire and that there is no time for an emergency landing. For unknown reasons, there are only four parachutes in the plane. I order my copilot to put on his parachute and to assist the three passengers to put on theirs. I then order my copilot and the three passengers to jump out of the plane. Not long after they exit the plane, it bursts into flames, and I am incinerated. My copilot and three passengers glide safely to the ground with their parachutes. *Was my motive to save their lives altruistic? Maybe I really wanted the last parachute but was too shy or too guilt ridden to ask for it. I have to put the welfare of my passengers before my own, right? Maybe I was thinking it would be spectacular to go down in flames while my passengers survive and have all this commemorated in a movie that would tout me as a hero. Maybe I knew it would make me feel good to give all the parachutes to the other people so they could be saved and return to their families. Maybe I was fearless about death and really didn't care at all that I didn't get a parachute (or that I gave them all to other people) because I believed I would go to heaven if I died in the plane crash.*

While altruism has the ultimate goal of increasing another person's welfare and egoism has the ultimate goal of increasing one's own welfare,[10] there *is* ethical room for unintended benefits to one's own welfare. Some might consider altruism, which includes the unintended benefits to one's own welfare, a *special* form of egoism because these unintended benefits emerge from within the helper/giver. They are not benefits bestowed from some external source, such as the person who received the help. In the airplane example above, the internal benefits could include knowing I did "the right thing," feeling good about giving away the parachutes, and not feeling guilty because I didn't take one of the parachutes. With the empathy-altruism hypothesis, the empathetic concern felt for a person in need produces an altruistic motivation to attend to the need. While doing so, however, there are three other possible results. In addition to the needy person getting aid, the helper may experience some benefits: 1) reduction of personal distress (the feelings that motivated the helper to respond to the need), 2) avoiding feeling guilty for not helping or avoiding having others think negatively because help was not given, and 3) gain of personal rewards, such as praise, recognition, and pride. These three items were not the *ultimate* goal of the helper; rather, the ultimate goal was to improve the welfare of the other person. Empathetic concern produces altruistic motivations, and these are not ethically marred by the unintended positive consequences to the helper.

ALTRUISM AND LIVING ORGAN DONATION

While altruism is ideally foundational to the concept of Good Samaritan donation, many transplant centers are frightened. One of the reasons for their fear is that many take a "black-and-white" approach to altruism. If they see gray ("benefits to the donor"), they have ethical distress that the donation might not be altruistically motivated (pure). As shown, not all indirect benefits to a helper mar the altruistic nature of the gift. In the setting of living organ donation, careful psychological screening of candidates is needed to ensure that potential donors are not donating to attempt to heal their own personal problems (e.g., to make amends for past misdeeds or to attempt to earn the respect of a relative). If that is their *ultimate* goal, they are not ethically suitable living donor candidates. If living organ donation is a form of personal psychological exploration, that too is not the appropriate ultimate goal. The ultimate goal must be to improve the recipient's welfare.

Another fear that transplant centers often have is the belief that a person who gives a living organ to a stranger "must be crazy." Organ vending is another anxiety among transplant center personnel. No transplant center wants to be caught in a scandal involving donors selling their organs (*why would they give their organs to strangers with "no strings attached"?*) They also don't want the headache and bad press of dealing with donors with psychological problems, and they have concerns about the ability of these individuals to give informed consent (not to mention concerns about donor motivations). These parallel fears have resulted in many U.S. transplant centers not permitting Good Samaritan donation. Further, some countries have banned the practice entirely (e.g., Egypt and France). California is the first U.S. state to have a living donor registry. Signed into law in 2010, the regulation creates the California Living Donor Registry to formally facilitate Good Samaritan donation.[11] This registry allows individuals to sign up, professing their desire to be a living kidney donor. In the future, the registry intends to expand to include other living donations (e.g., liver).

When Good Samaritan organ donation emerged in the United States in the 1960s, researchers were aware of the concerns and sought to systematically explore them as well as the motivations of these donors. The first such study was published in 1971 and included data from nine kidney donors.[12] As part of this study, transplant center teams were asked about their opinion of "living, unrelated" donors. Of the fifty-four transplant centers polled, only eleven were allowing this type of donation. The prevailing opinion was that of distrust of their motivations as well as their "mental health." Other feelings expressed were that these donors are "influenced by subliminal forces" and are "screwballs."[13] Donor motivations were felt to be based on "guilt," "atonement," and "a perverted sense of goodness."[14] Exploration of the donor data found that in only one case was the motivation described as "selfish."[15] Specifically, the donor (a former nurse) decided to donate as an attempt to "reconstruct [her] broken life."[16] She responded to a newspaper plea for donation to a stranger. As she told the researchers,[17] "[Donation was the] only good thing I ever did. I'm better for it. . . . It makes me forget the bad things of my past." This donor had a criminal history that included jail time as well as prior drug addiction and social isolation. While donation initially made her feel good, when the recipient died two months after transplant, the donor emotionally decompensated and was temporarily admitted to a state psychiatric facility. After discharge, she reported that she felt she had benefited from the aftermath and that the donation was a "wholesome" experience.[18] In retrospect, the researchers pose that this individual would not be accepted as a donor under today's standards because of "antisocial character disorder."[19]

For the other eight donors, several professed altruistic motivations that focused on the concept of "giving another life."[20] For those who responded to media pleas for donations, the "overwhelming reason" was to help someone in distress or to give them life. More than half the candidates who were screened as potential donors to these patients had a childhood that was disrupted and destabilized, enabling them to identify with the recipient's life situation. All nine donors experienced hospitalizations and follow-up periods that were without serious medical complications. These researchers concluded, "without hesitation," that these donations should be allowed to occur as a formal practice at transplant centers under strict protocols for candidate screening.[21]

Other researchers have followed in the steps of Sadler et al. and reported interesting findings, several of which are similar to our own. Henderson et al. identified the following motivations: 1) the desire to improve the quality of life of another person, 2) the desire to improve one's self-esteem, and 3) the desire to make a personal statement against one's family.[22] Several researchers have reported religion as the motivator[23] as well as a prior history of blood or

Table 1.1.   Donor Primary Motivations

Donor (Quantity)	Primary Motivation
7	Help another person/alleviate suffering
3	Empathy for the sick person
2	Love of science/impressed by surgical technology
2	Prior blood/marrow donor (organ donation was logical next step)
2	Save a life
2	Physically up to the task and could think of no reason to not donate
1	The world needs this behavior—it is the opposite of selfishness
1	God directed the individual to donate
1	Give back to society
1	Spiritual commandment, moral imperative to donate

marrow donation as precipitating organ donation as a next step.[24] Table 1.1 summarizes the primary motivations reported by the twenty-two donors we interviewed. Reviewing these data finds that twenty of twenty-two donors reported an altruistic motivation for donation as their primary drive. The most common theme, "wanting to help," is consistent with research results from a group studying Good Samaritan kidney donation in the Netherlands.[25] For our two individuals who reported a love of science and being impressed by living donor surgery technology, both also reported a desire to help others ("Why wouldn't I do this?" and "giving is just important to me. I don't even miss the other kidney. To just be able to give them life without having to be tied down to machines"). None voiced a motivation based on selfishness, guilt, atonement, "a perverted sense of goodness," or "craziness." The donor team's screening process was clearly robust at all fifteen participating hospitals.

Altruism is a values-driven concept. The values we hold help steer us toward particular activities. Clearly, not everyone is willing to be an organ donor (even if they are clinically able), so it is important to explore what underlies this unique volunteerism. To do this, we administered a validated survey called the Volunteer Motivation Inventory[26] to twenty-one of the donors in this book project (one donor was lost to follow-up). They were asked to read forty-four standardized statements of motivations for volunteering. The donors then ranked each statement on a scale of 1 to 5 to indicate how strongly they agreed (5) or disagreed (1) with the statement. These statements were coded for ten different motivational categories, including Values (importance of helping others), Recognition (being recognized for their contribution), Reciprocity ("what goes around comes around"), Self-Esteem (to improve one's self-worth and self-esteem), Reactivity (to heal and address past or current issues), Understanding (to improve the individual's understanding of themselves), and Protective (to reduce personal negative feelings such as guilt). Example statements from the survey are listed below:

> *I volunteer because I am concerned about those less fortunate than myself.*
> *I volunteer because I believe you receive what you put out in the world.*
> *Volunteering helps me deal with some of my own problems.*

Each donor's survey was then scored using a mathematical formula. The results assigned a numerical value between 1 and 5 for each of the ten motivational categories. The category with the highest score reflects the motivation of greatest importance to the donor, whereas the category with the lowest score reflects the motivation of least importance. For fifteen of twenty-one (71 percent) donors, Values (helping others just for the sake of helping) was the top-ranking score, noting that three of these donors had tie scores with Values and either Reciprocity or Understanding. The average Values score for these donors was 4.3 (1–5 scale). Overall, this was consistent with the verbal interview statements about motivations for donating.

NEIGHBORLINESS, EMPATHY, AND TRUST

Returning to the foundation of the word "altruism" (Italian *altrui*, "somebody else") and the historical concept of a Good Samaritan, the theme of *neighbor* emerges. Indeed, when Jesus was telling the story of the Good Samaritan, it was in response to a query about who is to be considered a neighbor.[27] We also explored this concept with the donors we interviewed. Specifically, we asked two true-or-false questions: 1) *All humans belong to one family* and 2) *As a child I sought out ways to correct injustice.* We obtained responses from twenty-one of twenty-two donors for both questions (one donor was lost to follow-up). Nearly all (twenty of twenty-one) believe that all humans belong to one family and thus are "our neighbors." We interpreted "correcting injustice as a child" as a form of reaching out to neighbors. This type of behavior was evidenced by thirteen of twenty-one (62 percent) donors. Our results appear to show that altruism, neighborliness, and Good Samaritan behavior are interconnected concepts.

As discussed earlier, empathy, the ability to understand and share the feelings of another, is also an interconnected concept. This is because "another" is a "neighbor," as all humanity belongs to "one family," according to twenty of twenty-one of our surveyed donors. As reported in table 1.1, we found empathy to be the second most reported response from our donors when asked directly, *What was your primary motivator?* Additionally, we explored the concept of empathy by asking the following true-or-false question: *As a child, I was troubled if I saw another child being bullied or humiliated or if I saw violence in cartoons.* Nearly all

our donors agreed with the statement (eighteen of twenty-one), indicating a relationship to the concept of empathy as well as "another" (neighbor). Behavioral
psychologists have well studied these ideas and know that empathy is not merely
taking in another person's feelings but also making a response to the person in
some way (either emotionally or with a "prosocial" act).[28] When people volunteer as organ donors, they take on responsibility for the welfare of others out of
concern for them. Both volunteering and empathizing are not passive behaviors.
Indeed, 62 percent of our donors sought to correct injustice as a child.

In another attempt to explore the concept of empathy, we asked our
twenty-two Good Samaritan donors to complete a written survey called the
Interpersonal Reactivity Index.[29] This is a validated instrument developed
by psychologist Mark Davis, and it has been used by empathy researchers
for more than twenty years. The survey is brief, containing only twenty-
eight situational items in which respondents rank their answers on a scale
of 1 ("does not describe me well") to 5 ("describes me very well"). As
examples, two items from the survey are *I often have tender, concerned feelings
for people less fortunate than me* and *When I see someone being taken advantage of,
I feel kind of protective toward them*. Overall, the survey explores the four dimensions of empathy: perspective taking (the donor's spontaneous attempts
to adopt the perspectives of others and see things from their point of view),
fantasy (the donor's tendency to identify with characters in movies, novels,
and other fictional scenarios), empathic concern (the donor's feelings of
warmth, compassion, and concern for others), and personal distress (the
donor's feelings of anxiety and discomfort that result from observing another's negative experience). Perspective taking and fantasy are considered
cognitive dimensions of empathy, whereas empathetic concern and personal
distress are considered emotional dimensions of empathy. Each dimension
is analyzed using a simple mathematical formula that results in a final score
ranging from 0 to 28.

Eighteen of twenty-two of our donors completed the survey. Of these,
twelve were men, and six were women. With regard to empathetic concern,
the average score was 24.9; perspective taking, 20.7; fantasy, 14.5; and personal
distress, 6.6. We found that there were no significant differences between men
and women donors, except in the category of personal distress. Specifically,
women donors were approximately two and a half times more likely to experience personal distress (anxiety, discomfort, fear, and apprehension) when observing another person's negative experience (e.g., an emergency). Fourteen
of eighteen donors ranked empathic concern as the highest-scoring dimension
of the four categories, while two donors had this category tied with perspective taking for their highest score. For the remaining two donors who did not
rank empathic concern as their highest score, both gave perspective taking
top rank. Overall, our survey results are consistent with the general field of
empathy research; that is, greater perspective-taking ability is associated with

greater feelings of empathic concern for others. This is because empathy is an other-oriented activity. The connection to Good Samaritan organ donation is obvious, as these individuals have the ability to turn their attention outward, away from themselves, toward others who are experiencing distress.

The concept of trust is also inexplicably linked to neighborliness and altruism. This is because trust cannot occur in isolation but rather involves *another* party (neighbor). In its form as a noun, the word "trust" involves taking on responsibility for someone (or something), as in trusteeship. As a verb, "trust" involves having faith or confidence in a person or thing. Personality psychologists have studied these concepts and determined that we tend to feel responsible for the people we trust and tend to feel bad when they experience problems originating without their control (illness).[30] Trusting people are also more likely to give these individuals helpful services.[31] In the setting of organ donation, these are the neighbors whom Good Samaritans respond to when hearing about or seeing their affliction, especially those cases involving childhood genetic disorders such as cystic fibrosis and biliary atresia. Indeed, nineteen of twenty-one (90 percent) of our donors informed us that they consider themselves to be "generally trusting of others."

According to psychologists, people considered to be "trusting" have faith in the basic decency of humanity.[32] We confirmed this concept as well when we asked our donors the following true-or-false question: *In general, the world is good.* Sixteen of twenty-one (76 percent) responded with the belief that the world, in general, *is* good (even though at times people behave "badly"). It's unclear if this "basic decency" is related to religious or spiritual beliefs about personhood or human dignity, as these require deep theological and philosophical deconstructions. However, the concept of basic human decency does have input from religious principles even if there is no agreement as to its foundation. Looking again to our donors, we noted that fifteen of twenty-one (71 percent) reported that religious beliefs or spirituality contribute to their desire to help others. Notably, all our donors who professed a religious affiliation were either Protestant or Catholic. While we did not have any Jewish donors in our group, our sample size was small. We know that these donors do exist, as does a unique website to promote Good Samaritan organ donations from the Jewish community.[33] In general, psychologists have determined that "frequent churchgoers volunteer more than non-religious people, regardless of their religious faith or denomination."[34] We speculate that this could be due to scripture, tenets, and practices that pertain to compassion, benevolence, and service to others.[35] In a subsequent chapter, we take a deeper look at the concept of service to others while exploring the patterns of such service in Good Samaritan organ donors.

Fred: A Real-Life Superhero

$\mathcal{M}$any marketing executives get up for work in the morning, put on a business suit, grab their briefcase, and head out the door. Fred, however, is not your "normal" businessman. Many would call him Superman because he gave one of his kidneys to a stranger. In fact, his daily work uniform is a cape and leotards that make him resemble the "Man of Steel."[1] A Rotarian,[2] Fred truly believes in "Service above Self," and there is hardly a better example than Good Samaritan organ donation.

Rotarians are known for their volunteer work, and many participate in health care–related projects, such as polio eradication (PolioPlus)[3] or cleft lip and palate repair (Rotaplast).[4] There is even a Rotary project dedicated to providing free living kidney transplants to needy patients in developing countries (Lifeplant).[5] When Rotarians consider taking up an endeavor, they subject it to the Four Way Test: 1) Is it the *truth*? 2) Is it *fair* to all concerned? 3) Will it build *goodwill* and *better friendships*? and 4) Will it be *beneficial* to all concerned? Good Samaritan organ donation passed the test when Fred examined the concept closely.

When Fred is not wearing his cape-and-leotard costume to promote the benefits of credit union membership, he looks a lot like mild-mannered newspaper reporter Clark Kent (the civilian version of Superman). In fact, when Fred (the youngest of four children) was growing up, he wanted to be a newspaper reporter just like his father. Interestingly, a medical theme was also present in his family. His mother was director of respiratory therapy at a hospital, and his sister is an oncology nurse. Thus, Fred was not completely unfamiliar with the medical profession when he entered the operating room to give away a kidney.

At forty-three years of age, Fred's donation journey began when he watched a news story on television about an individual who gave a kidney to a coworker. Fred was intrigued and thought that there was no reason he couldn't do the same. Even though he didn't know anyone who needed a kidney, he still wanted to give one of his away. "There's gotta be someone out there that needs one!"[6] And his motivation for giving was clear and simple: saving a life. The next morning, he called the two transplant hospitals in his area to inquire about donation. Even his fear of needles did not deter him. Within a few weeks, he was at Hartford Hospital in Connecticut starting his medical and psychosocial evaluations.

Not far away was a stranger, undergoing her routine dialysis treatment. A single mother with three children, Pam's kidneys were devastated by a genetic condition called polycystic kidney disease (PKD). This disorder causes the production of cysts inside the kidney that causes the kidney to swell. The result is high blood pressure and infections. Additionally, patients with PKD have increased production of the hormone erythropoietin. This leads to a problematic overproduction of red blood cells. Cysts that are painful, infected, bleeding, or causing an obstruction may need to be drained, or the kidney may need to be surgically removed. Currently, there are no treatments that prevent the cysts from forming or enlarging. Patients rely on dialysis for temporary relief or kidney transplantation for their cure. In addition to the burdens of dialysis, Pam had endured abscesses and repeated hospitalizations. A transplant would be a miracle for her.

Besides the routine medical consultations and tests, Fred was assessed by a social worker and a psychiatrist to verify that his motives were altruistic and that his mental health was sound. Certainly his volunteer work with Rotary and his longtime history of blood donation were indicators of a pattern of prosocial behavior. He also had absolutely no intention of selling his kidney to anyone. It was a gift. His wife, Robin, supported his choice to donate but, like most spouses, had concerns about the potential future need of a kidney by a family member. Fred had already thought about that concept carefully and ruled it out. He honestly could not foresee that need and desired to continue with his donation plans. When he received official medical and psychosocial clearance, his intended recipient was informed of the good news. At the time, she was hooked to a dialysis machine when her doctor told her that a donor had been found. She was overjoyed. She had lost her father to kidney disease, but *she* was going to get a second chance at life.

But who was this donor? A stranger was coming from out of the blue to give her a kidney? According to Fred, the intended recipient learned his identity a few days before surgery. It happened by accident. The local television station had interviewed Fred about his upcoming surgery and mentioned the place and date of the donation. Pam's friends were watching that news story and called her, talked about it, and, like detectives, put all the pieces together. Unless it was a coincidence, Pam was going to get Fred's kidney in a few days.

Indeed, two days after surgery, Pam and Fred met at the hospital as they recovered. To this day, they are close friends, and Fred refers to her as his "kidney caretaker."[7] For Fred, it was not the act of donation that was important to him but rather the fact that donation could save another person's life. As Fred says bluntly, "You're not using your other kidney so don't be greedy."[8] And while Pam thinks Fred is her hero, Fred does not think of himself that way at all. For him, organ donation was no different that helping someone cross the street.[9] It's just another form of helping, something that he was able to do and something that he encourages other people to do as well ("anybody can do it".[10])

Fred is very satisfied with his donation experience. He suffered no complications other than a minor allergic reaction to medical adhesive tape. He even lost weight (as did several of our other Good Samaritan donors). Hoping to be able to save another life, Fred recently pursued clinical testing to be a living liver donor; however, blood tests revealed a risk for abnormal blood clotting, so he was declined as a candidate.

Fred's superhero costume now includes a green "Donate Life" wristband. Wherever he goes, he can promote credit union membership *and* organ donation. And when he's not doing that, he can be found sitting in his hot tub smoking a cigar or carousing with his two dogs, Oki and Macks. He's just a normal guy, not a hero (well, maybe Pam's hero).

• 3 •

Josie: Crisis Control

$\mathcal{J}$osie is a unique Good Samaritan donor. Notably, she is one of only a very few Asian American living donors in the United States. In 2009, only 3.4 percent of living donors in the United States were Asian American (most, 70 percent, were white).[1] In addition, Josie hates needles. Prior to her kidney donation, she had never had surgery before, and she was very fearful of the pain that would befall her. She also worried about the risk of dying during donation as well as the unknowns of the recovery process. But Josie is someone who can step up to the plate when needed. And this is just what she did in 2008.[2]

Josie and Allan have been a couple for seventeen years. They met at their first job after graduating from college. She is a personnel recruiter, and he is an application engineer for a semiconductor manufacturer. For many years, Allan had progressive kidney disease, but he tried not to let it slow him down. He enjoyed a lifestyle of scuba diving, golf, hiking, and trips to out-of-the-ordinary places like Tibet. But when his illness advanced and he developed end-stage kidney failure requiring dialysis, action was needed.

Josie has a pattern of responding in times of crises. When both of her parents were diagnosed with cancer and her four siblings could not take charge of the situation, she did. And when her husband was faced with a six- to eight-year wait for a kidney transplant (or endure the burdens of continued dialysis), she stepped up for that too. At thirty-nine years of age, she offered a kidney to him but was not an immunological match, so she agreed to a kidney swap involving another incompatible pair. The plan was for the two incompatible pairs to be shuffled to create two compatible pairs, but a few hours before surgery, there was a complication with the other donor–recipient pair, and all four surgeries (two donations, two transplants) were canceled. Josie had passed all the medical and psychosocial screenings and came within hours of kidney donation. Josie and Allan checked out of the hospital and left town for a few days to recover from the shock of it all.

Devastated but not defeated, Josie continued to advocate for her husband, and she joined Stanford University Medical Center's (Palo Alto, California) first kidney chain. Using unique computer software, the National Kidney Registry[3] assembled the chain of compatible matches within only a few weeks of their database enrollment. As part of this chain, Josie gave one of her kidneys to a stranger, and a stranger gave a kidney to her husband. Josie's recipient was in New York, so her kidney was removed, packed in ice, and flown across the United States. In total, the chain consisted of four hospitals, three donors, and three recipients.[4]

Josie's fears about postoperative pain were put to rest when she received a patient-controlled analgesia device at her hospital bedside. These are small machines that contain pain medication, which is directly administered by the patient when the patient presses a button on a handheld wand. The medication drips down thin cables of tubing through a needle in the patient's vein. Computer software in the machine functions to ensure that only safe doses of medication are delivered, preventing an overdose. Pain never became a problem for Josie as she was recuperating from donation, and she raves about the excellent care the Stanford team provided her. Josie recovered well and had no complications.

Interestingly, before entering the chain program, Josie's husband had considered multiple listing. This is a practice in which patients get wait listed at multiple hospitals in order to increase their odds of access to a deceased donor organ. But both he and Josie knew that the survival rates from transplants using living donor organs were better than those using deceased donor organs. In addition, multiple listing adds complexity to the transplant process because of extra expenses (e.g., travel) and logistical matters (e.g., the distance between the patient and transplant center must be manageable so that the patient can arrive at the hospital quickly when the organ is ready for transplant). While traveling to explore their options for multiple listing, they received the call that a match had been found via the chain mechanism. Josie didn't hesitate. They headed back to Stanford. "It was a no-brainer."[5]

Josie and her husband have returned to their normal life of daily three-mile walks, golf, tennis, restaurant hopping, and international travel. While her lifestyle has not changed, Josie says that she "appreciates things more,"[6] especially her good health. She is very thankful that her husband no longer requires dialysis, and she values the concept of chain donation because multiple people can be assisted through the help of individual strangers linking together, taking patients off the organ waiting list by way of their organ gifts.

So far, Josie has not met the recipient of her kidney, but she would like to know who the person is. Even if she never meets the individual, she does have interest in knowing about the person. To date, she has not received a thank-you letter from the recipient or the recipient's family, and she does not know if the individual is alive or dead, healthy or ill. While these matters are discussed with potential donors during the candidate screening process, actually facing the realities of these concepts can be difficult.

Is Josie still afraid of surgery? You bet, but she has no regrets and would repeat her decision to donate if given the opportunity. She describes her scar as "big" and "dark," but she says it doesn't bother her. She encourages others to be living donors and is always ready to answer people's questions about the topic.

· 4 ·

Matt: Making Amends

Where was the man with all the tattoos? He had sent photos of himself for easy recognition. Some of the images were of the tattoos he has all over his body, so the perception was of a man stepping out of a Harley-Davidson advertisement. But the man who appeared at the rainy Pennsylvania train station was just the opposite. He was conservatively dressed, and he could have kept casting directors busy for hours with roles in home improvement commercials. In a nearby hotel lobby, he explained his life history and what motivated his desire to give a kidney to a stranger.[1]

The most significant feature of Matt's childhood was his shyness. Now, covered in tattoos, his arms, back, and chest is a mural of his life—and his life has been eventful. There are designs representing his years working in a group home for kids with psychiatric disorders, his six years as a fisherman in Alaska, his fifty-two-day bicycle trip from Virginia Beach to San Diego, and his travels to Mexico during his six months off from his fishing job. When asked about the tattoos, he says, "It's a way of telling the world who I am, and if they don't like it, they can stay away. I'm more comfortable with 'counterculture' people. The tattoos keep the judgmental people away."[2] That perhaps is the way he's learned to cover his extreme shyness and to protect himself from hurt and humiliation.

Matt, so shy he couldn't speak in class, managed, when he was eleven, to get up the courage to try out for the basketball team. He was not one of the school's shining stars, and he and the other "losers"[3] were last to be interviewed by the coach. While the coach wasn't looking, the "jocks" pulled down the pants of the kids waiting to be interviewed. The coach was furious and rebuked them. Cowering, Matt left the gym. By the time he was twelve, he had become a drug addict and alcoholic.

27

Matt was born to middle-class Catholic parents in Reading, Pennsylvania. He has a twin sister ("She did everything right—I did everything wrong"[4]) and a younger brother who is bipolar and a recovering drug addict. Matt took over responsibility for him after he got multiple DUIs and wrecked two cars. "He was a handful and my folks couldn't control him. I could."[5] Matt feels some responsibility for the addiction. "I was his big brother—he wanted to be like me."[6] His brother eventually moved in with Matt and has been with him for three years. Matt took him to specialists who treated his bipolar disorder, got him into Narcotics Anonymous, and is able to say with pride and certainty, "He's my best friend."[7] Now a self-confident forty-year-old, Matt is tall and athletic and plays basketball regularly. He's come a long way from the miserable, terrified teenager who kept himself in a drug and alcoholic haze until he was nineteen.

Matt's decision to be a Good Samaritan organ donor is the direct result of his background. As he told us, "I think my upbringing had the most profound effect on my deciding to have the surgery."[8] His father (a social worker) and his mother (a nurse) instilled in him a sense of responsibility for those less fortunate. And despite—or perhaps because of—a troubled childhood and adolescence, he has sensitivity to the needs of others and the desire to help them. He may even have a desire to make amends for the unhappiness he caused his family over the years. After watching a television program about Good Samaritan donation, he was intrigued, and his helping instinct took over. Being an occupational therapist, he is no stranger to the clinical setting. "In the hospital we have a lot of patients with kidney disease and a lot of patients on dialysis, so I know that's a huge issue. I saw a program on TV a couple of years ago about a woman who was an anonymous kidney donor, and the thought always interested me. You know, you can live a normal healthy life with one kidney, so why not? Why not give the other one to someone who needs it? And I'm a good candidate—I'm young and healthy."[9]

In 2009, he gave a kidney to a stranger at New York Presbyterian Hospital. "I did a lot of research and wanted a hospital where they did a lot of transplants and where the outcomes were good."[10] After surgery, he didn't meet his recipient, a middle-aged woman originally from Barbados, as she was very sick. In fact, several months passed, and he had no contact at all from her. He was sad but not discouraged, as his donation was with no strings attached. And he didn't need any validation from others (including the recipient) that his act was honorable. Then suddenly, he got a phone call.[11] On the other end of the phone was a hospital social worker informing Matt that the recipient wanted to meet him.

Matt and his recipient met at a restaurant in New York. He brought his wife, and she brought her son. The number of coincidences that followed is amazing. The recipient has the same (rare) first name as Matt's twin sister. The recipient is a nurse, just like Matt's wife and mother. And Matt and the recipient's son share the same birth date (month and day). No wonder Matt and his recipient bonded instantly: they share so much in common, not to mention his kidney.

Matt has recovered from donation with no side effects and tells us, "Sometimes I forget that I even had the surgery."[12] He must have forgotten when he participated in a 100-mile bicycle ride as a fund-raising effort for multiple sclerosis research. He also told us, "I am running and playing basketball . . . I am a few pounds lighter!"[13] Looking back, would Matt repeat his decision to donate? "Absolutely!"[14] And if someone else opens the door to the topic, he will tell them about it. He downplays his altruistic act and states that "it's not for everybody."[15] He is very reflective about the suffering in the world and has a lot of empathy for people in the position that his recipient was in before she was transplanted. Dialysis is a "difficult lifelong situation,"[16] but organ donation can change that.

II

DESTINED TO BE A DONOR

Constructs of Destiny

SERVING GOD

*A*ltruists serve the community with their volunteerism. However, an individual can serve both God and humanity (community) when there is an underlying spiritual or religious conviction. While the vast majority of our twenty-two Good Samaritan donors expressed religious or spiritual values, three believe that God was explicitly involved in their decision to donate. Similar findings have also been reported in medical literature. Psychiatrists David Dixon and Susan Abbey from Toronto General Hospital (Canada) published a case report about a Catholic man who wanted to donate a kidney to a member of his church whom he had never met but heard needed a transplant.[1] During his evaluation at the transplant center, the man informed clinicians that his motivation for donating stemmed from modeling the self-giving love of Jesus as well as Eucharistic activities of sharing the body (bread) and blood (wine). He also disclosed a history of physical abuse as a youth and problems with anger management and self-harm that were under control within recent years. Some members of the donor team had strong opinions against allowing the man to donate. Among other things, these opinions were based on the view that a religious motivation for donation was pathological.[2]

Exploring further, the "pathology" was divided into two forms: religious psychosis and religion-inspired guilt. Some at the transplant center also wondered whether the man could have really cleaned up his life through religion, as he had claimed. *Could religion really produce psychological health in someone who had experienced so much life turmoil?* Some felt that both his donation offer and his psychological recovery were not sound because they had religious underpinnings. It seemed that religion had pathologized the man, labeling him as suspect and unfit. Clearly, unfairness is found in judgments made by way of religious bias and prejudicial generalizations. The end result is the potential to turn away capable altruistic donors. We believe that religious motivations for organ donation should not be a categorical exclusion, nor should they be termed pathological. Each potential donor should be evaluated as a unique individual who has many features, not just religious or spiritual ones. But what do you do when a congregation lines up at your front door with the desire to donate as an explicit religious tenet?

The Mayo Clinic in Rochester, Minnesota, has had unique experience with religiously motivated kidney donors. In 2003, the Mayo Clinic performed a donor nephrectomy on David McKay, leader of the small religious sect Jesus Christians.[3] At the time, they did not know this vocational information, and he had passed all medical and psychosocial screenings. After his successful donation, six more Jesus Christians asked to come to the Mayo Clinic to be kidney donors. According to this sect, organ donation is "a natural and practical application of Jesus' command to love our neighbour."[4] The Mayo Clinic, however, was ethically troubled by their en masse request. It was not that Mayo believed that altruism couldn't be motivated by religion; rather, the clinic worried that the donor candidates might not be autonomous and free of coercion (by their religious leader). In fact, when two of six candidates were evaluated by the Mayo Clinic team, both expressed financial, spiritual, and social dependence on their sect leader (who advocated kidney donation on religious grounds). This was a red flag for the Mayo Clinic, which felt that such facts potentially caused coercion, and both individuals were declined as donor candidates. Additionally, no further Jesus Christian candidates were considered. We attempted to include Jesus Christian donors in our interview pool; however, their leader discouraged his members from interacting with us. To date, nearly half the Jesus Christians sect has donated kidneys around the world (about twenty donations so far).[5]

Elsewhere, physicians reported the ethically complex case of an ordained Buddhist monk who wanted to donate a kidney to a stranger.[6] Her motivation to donate came from her religious faith, which promoted helping humanity. What made her donation request ethically problematic was not the religious-based motivation but rather that she wanted to selectively direct her donation to an individual who was not involved in a specific type of activity, namely, killing (e.g., hunter, angler, or soldier). She also preferred that her donation be allocated to a racial or ethnic minority patient, but she did not view this as an absolute requirement. The monk passed all medical and psychosocial screenings and was permitted to donate; however, it was decided that she could not place vocational, racial, or ethnic restrictions on the donation, as this would be a form of discrimination. The monk agreed to the hospital's terms, and her donation was without complication. In her thank-you letter to the hospital, she remarked on her religious convictions and hoped that her donation would be used for the "greater good" (potentially spawning more donations to save more lives).[7]

Three of our Good Samaritan donors expressed that God was instrumental in their decision to donate. In the coming chapters, you will read their full stories, but here we will give you a brief synopsis. Dave gave a lung lobe to a teenager with cystic fibrosis after taking a walk on a California beach and hearing God speak to him in a voice he couldn't ignore.[8] According to Dave, following God's plan was essential because in the past, he had a specific incident of disregarding the voice of God, and the consequences were dire. He was not going to make the same mistake twice. He felt that God's plan involved both himself and a specifically identified patient (Matthew); thus, it was critical that he carry out the exact plan and not deviate from it. As Dave states, he had several "God confirmations"[9] throughout the predonation process that validated that he was following His will. Although he has reduced lung capacity now (because he has less lung tissue), he has no regrets about donating and would "do it again in a heartbeat."

Cheryl, a Good Samaritan kidney donor in Maryland, had a similar story.[10] She had read a newspaper article about a man on dialysis and felt empathy toward him. According to Cheryl, after reading the article, she felt God speaking to her, telling her, "This is what I want you to do!" Reading the article, Cheryl thought, "Oh, I'm made for this man!" Even though the transplant hospital was not as enthusiastic as Cheryl, because she and the patient were not emotionally related, Cheryl persisted so that she could satisfy her calling. Under her terms, she created a "relationship" that set the foundation that started the cascade of events toward donation. Her hospital stay was thirty-six hours and she resumed driving her car another forty-eight hours later. For Cheryl, "It was meant to happen. It was His [God's] plan for me."

Max, a grocery store department manager and Good Samaritan kidney donor, told us, "God had been tugging at my heart to do something. It had been something in my heart for a while."[11] He was already registered to be an organ and tissue donor after death, but a pay stub donation challenge triggered Max to take action. Accepting his employer's challenge, everything fell into place. As Max states, "Everything was happening the way I felt it was supposed to happen. I knew it was just planned because I just kept getting more and more peace all the way through."[12]

ANOTHER VIEW OF DESTINY

Not all perspectives of the concept of destiny are based on God. For some, destiny can be part of the order of the universe or some other construction.

Even people who believe in God, attend church, and read the Bible or other religious text might opt for a view of destiny that is based not on a divine preordination but rather on a series or cascade of events of their free will. In a subsequent chapter, you will read Jeff's full donation story, but here we present the key points that pertain to his "destiny" to be a donor. Jeff considers himself a spiritual but not religious person.[13] He finds truth in many religions but does not use a particular one to guide his daily living. His life has taken many turns, including his loss of eyesight as a child, progressive hearing loss, and assuming the oversight of his cognitively disabled brother. But amid all this, which some would call harm or chaos, Jeff seems to find order. In his own words, "I wanted to fulfill my destiny to the greatest eventuality possible. . . . I felt like it [living donation] was given to me to do."[14] Even with his own clinical and personal challenges, Jeff could not come up with a reason to not pursue donation and even viewed it as a moral imperative for him personally. After donation, Jeff endured five months of chronic pain and nausea, which were treated with various medications, herbs, and hydrotherapy. He has no regrets about donating and says that "great good resulted."[15]

Jack, another Good Samaritan kidney donor whom we will profile fully in a subsequent chapter, lives about eighteen miles from Jeff (and they have since met and become friends). Jack is a strong believer in fate. He wasn't even fearful about donating because, as he stated, "I believe that whatever happens is going to happen. It was almost predetermined what was going to take place in my life. Because of believing so heavily in fate and not having control over anything, I really thought that everything was going to be okay."[16] Jack believes that his life has purpose: "I feel that's why I was put on earth, is to make a difference in making life better for an individual or a group of individuals."[17] Looking back, Jack has no regrets about his decision to donate. He suffered no complications and terms it a positive experience "from start to finish."[18]

IS ALTRUISM INNATE?

With evidence that some altruists feel that their behavior was destined, *could it be that altruism is innate or genetic? Are some humans born with (or without) these tendencies?* Studies in nonhuman animals, as well as human twin pairs, has led many to conclude that altruism does have a genetic basis. In the world of nonhuman animals, the honeybee is perhaps the most familiar example. The honeybee makes an altruistic sacrifice of his or her life in order to promote the life of the colony. Specifically, when threatened, the honeybee will sting and leave its sharp, angled dagger in the victim. Detachment of the stinger causes the bee's death because vital portions of the bee's body are additionally ripped away. The bee has protected the hive but sacrificed his or her own life in doing so. Additionally, worker bees that are sick are known to remove themselves from the hive (their source of safety and food) so that they don't contaminate the colony.[19] Several species of termites employ a similar suicidal altruism. When threatened, they use a process called autothysis, which involves secreting a sticky substance from their skin after the termite self-detonates (ruptures itself). Ants who try to invade the termite colony become entangled in a sticky mess of goop and dead termites.[20] Nonsuicidal altruism is also evident in nonhuman animals. For example, dolphins have been known to swim alongside sick or injured mammals in order to provide them protection and help them to the surface when needed.[21]

In humans, it seems that there would be a genetic purpose to altruism: promotion of our species. In fact, researchers are exploring whether there is a genetic connection between dopamine (a neurotransmitter in the brain) and altruism. Dopamine is associated with the pleasure and reward system of the brain, providing feelings of enjoyment and reinforcement that motivate individuals to proactively perform certain activities. Researchers in Germany hypothesize that a specific gene variant in the dopamine system caused more altruistic activity in their sample of research subjects.[22] But even if there is not an "altruism gene," there may well be genes that ultimately get activated (by the environment or other factors) and that wire the brain for empathy and caring as potential feeling and behavioral options. In fact, magnetic resonance imaging studies have shown that there are some areas of the brain that are specifically linked to altruistic behavior, and these areas of the brain are notably active in empathetic situations.[23] If there are many of these neural paths in the brain, it would seem that there would be more opportunities for helping behavior (if the person chooses to act on his or her emotions and feelings). Being prewired for altruism and then nurtured by early life events and parental modeling, for example, could promote an altruistic life.[24] Replicating this over and over through generations could continue to produce humans with altruistic tendencies.[25]

Some researchers who study children and their growth and development pose that altruism is evident at a very early age.[26] They argue that altruistic behavior appears so early in human life (infancy) that it could not have been taught, and neither could babies be rationally making altruistic choices in response to a moral duty (whether it be personal or universal).[27] An infant brain cannot process concepts such as moral codes or principles. Nonetheless, even infants exhibit altruistic behavior in which they don't take into account who receives their help (a relative, friend, or stranger), if their help will give them a reward, or if their help will improve their reputation. Perhaps as children grow older and have more life experiences, they become more discriminate about their altruistic behavior (to whom and what they give).

In the setting of living donation, an altruistic motivation is converted to an altruistic behavior. With our Good Samaritans, we observed a tendency for a quick decision when it came to their pronouncement to be a donor. They did not need someone to convince them to donate, and they did not "hem and haw" or vacillate. This does not mean that they did not make an informed decision; rather, they had a rapid and irrevocable internal conviction of the need to mobilize and act in an altruistic way to help a needy person. The informed consent process came later after receiving ample information about the procedure and its risks and benefits.

When we asked our twenty-two Good Samaritan donors how much time elapsed between deciding to donate and contacting a transplant hospital to inform them of the desire, nine (41 percent) indicated that as little as twenty-four hours had passed. Four of twenty-two (18 percent) indicated that two to four weeks had passed. Three donors waited one to four months. Six donors pondered their decision for a year or longer before contacting a transplant hospital to make plans for the evaluation and donation procedures. Looking closely at the data for the nine donors who made a quick decision (twenty-four hours or less), we observed that six of them (67 percent) ranked "values" with the highest score on the Volunteer Motivation Inventory survey.[28] Of those donors who waited a year or longer before contacting a transplant hospital with their decision, we observed that 67 percent of them also ranked "values" with the highest score on the Volunteer Motivation Inventory survey. As discussed earlier, high scores in the "values" theme equate to holding the belief that it is important to help others just for the sake of helping (without motivation for personal gain such as feeling good, recognition, or other rewards). Even though both groups of donors behaved very differently in terms of the time elapsed before contacting a transplant hospital, both groups shared the same motivational theme. They both helped for the same reason, but one group moved at a much slower pace from their altruistic value to their helping behavior. Many things can slow the pace (e.g., economic instability, relocation, spousal discord, and job and parenting responsibilities); nonetheless, for altruists, it seems that they are determined to carry out helping behaviors. *Maybe scientists are right when they pose a biological rationale for altruism. Maybe the brains of some people are wired for helping behaviors.*

Concepts of genetics, destiny, and fate require us to inject words of caution. Individuals may feel strongly that their life plan includes living organ donation; however, life circumstances may intervene and make donation unsafe or unadvisable (even if clinically safe). If this is the case, individuals should step back and accept the situation rather than make unwise choices that jeopardize their safety and welfare. Indeed, this is why the role of Independent Living Donor Advocate (ILDA) is so important.[29] All U.S. transplant centers have at least one ILDA (a regulatory requirement), and their role includes evaluation of the decision making of donor candidates. For example, if an individual wishes to be a donor but the idea is causing significant marital strife, the ILDA might recommend that the donation not occur (or that the spouses receive joint counseling before matters go farther). If an individual appears financially burdened and without means of social support yet is insistent on being a living donor, the ILDA would likely advise the donor team that the candidate be declined, at least temporarily, until his or her life is economically and socially enhanced so as to be more prepared for the donation experience. A candidate's life may need some stabilization before a significant event like donation occurs. The ILDA attempts to inject objectivity into donation decision making.

A subsequent chapter will explore how donor decision making can impact one's family. While the donor might be an altruist, not everyone in the family may share that philosophy. This can be a source of discord. For example, it might seem precarious for the sole breadwinner to put his life on the line for a stranger when he has a wife and three children at home to support. In addition, how do potential donors inform their young children of their pending surgery and the rationale for it? *Should they be informed?* Donors don't live in a vacuum. Their decisions do impact those closest to them.

· 6 ·

Dave: The Voice
on the Beach

$\mathcal{D}$ave is not someone you want banging on your front door at three in the morning. If your neighbor has a tunnel leading from the backyard playhouse to Mexico, Dave likely knows about it. If there is a house on the block with an unusually high electric bill, Dave likely knows about that too. This is no man to mess with unless you like cramped quarters, surly roommates, bologna sandwiches for lunch every day, and a uniform of horizontal stripes and flip-flops. You see, Dave is a U.S. Customs special agent who investigates narcotics smuggling, among other things. He is strong, and he is smart. And he has a heart of gold.

Dave grew up in the midwestern portion of the United States and has an identical twin.[1] His father was an X-ray technician and his mother a house-wife. As a child, his goal was to become a police officer, and he accomplished that and went farther, becoming a federal law enforcement special agent. His job requires him to have few fears and to be willing to lay his life on the line for others. Thus, it's no surprise that he was willing to give a lung lobe to save a child's life. Living lung lobe donation is risky, and few in the world have given lobes to strangers. And while the risk was present, even more present on Dave's mind was a memory from his past.

In 1991, when Dave was enrolled at the Federal Law Enforcement Training Center in Georgia, he arranged to have his fiancée, Kelly, fly in for a visit. Before her arrival, he had a feeling that something would go wrong, but he didn't call her and tell her his concern because he assumed that he was just being overly anxious. As the plane was about to land, a small internal voice told him that something was wrong with the plane, and, indeed, the plane crashed. All twenty-three passengers and crew on the twin turboprop aircraft, including his fiancée, a former senator, and an astronaut, were killed.[2] The

40

National Transportation Safety Board concluded that malfunction of the left-engine propeller control unit caused the plane to turn and then nose-dive on approach to Brunswick, Georgia.[3] Dave blames himself for ignoring his initial concern and not listening to that internal voice. He vowed never to make that life-altering mistake again.

In 2000, while driving back to San Diego after working an assignment in Los Angeles, Dave became drowsy and pulled off the Pacific Coast Highway at San Onofre. This stretch of beach is famous for its proximity to a strange-looking set of buildings (a nuclear power plant) and an expanse of waves that is paradise for surfers. Dave got out of his car and went for a walk along the shore in order to breathe some crisp sea air for refreshment and rejuvenation. He began skipping stones along the shore and thinking about his days at summer camp in Michigan. The 1899 hymn "I'll Go Where You Want Me to Go"[4] came to his mind and played on prominently. By the time Dave got back to his car, he knew that God wanted him to do something, but he didn't know what. He did know that he was going to listen *this* time!

The following evening he was watching television, and a story aired about a teenager with cystic fibrosis who needed a lung transplant to survive. Dave instantly knew that lung lobe donation was his mission. He looked at his wife, Rhonda, and announced, "That's me!"[5] The next morning, he called the television station and was referred to the hospital for a clinical evaluation. While he was a perfect match, the hospital was ethically distraught at the concept of Good Samaritan donation. The standard clinical practice at their facility was for the donor–recipient pair to be related either genetically or emotionally (e.g., friend, spouse, or colleague). But Dave was insistent. He informed the hospital that he had responded to the television plea and that he was *going* to be the donor. The hospital "grilled" him extensively during the psychosocial evaluation as part of their due diligence that his motivations were virtuous. To thwart possible negative reactions about his spirituality, Dave didn't tell the doctors about his divine directive to donate. He didn't want to be labeled as having some sort of religious pathology. He was already walking on eggshells with the transplant hospital, and a diagnosis like that could eliminate him as a donor.

Within a few days, Matt, the scrawny teenager who had been an avid surfer, received his new lungs: one lobe from Dave and another from a customer at the grocery store where Matt's mom worked.[6] Soon, Matt was back surfing his favorite California waves and traveling to exotic waters around the world. He grew several inches in height and added flesh to his thin frame. He even acquired for himself a new birthday, November 2, the day of his transplant. The living donor transplant extended Matt's life eight years, and during that time Dave was a witness to him about his faith and spirituality. In the years before Dave moved to the East Coast of the United States, he and Matt were often able to spend time together and Dave considered Matt part of his family. Dave also became part of Matt's family. Matt eventually required a retransplant and died shortly thereafter, but Dave knows that he obeyed the voice of God when he gave Matt a lung lobe. He has no regrets and would repeat his donation if he had the chance. When Dave is barreling down ski slopes, he has fond memories of Matt barreling through ocean waves.

Like many of the Good Samaritan donors we interviewed, Dave is a Christian. But neither Matt nor his family were religious, and it was baffling to him that they did not see what Dave saw: the hand of God in the donation. For Dave, the donation was not an act based on sentimental emotions or empathy; rather, it was a response to the call of God. And the donation could not have gone to just anyone because for Dave to honor God's will, the gift had to be directed to Matt.

Matt's family is still a special part of Dave's life, and he spends time with them whenever he returns to southern California on business trips. He also maintains contact with them via phone. The impact of the donation was likely very personal to Matt, and he likely had thoughts and emotions he never expressed. Had he more time on the planet, we might know more about his perception of concepts such as religion and spirituality. Instead, we are left knowing a boy who resumed life at his favorite place—the ocean—the same place where events all started for Dave, skipping stones and hearing a hymn.

• 7 •

Cheryl: The Game
Is on Hold Today

*C*heryl is a mass of contradictions.[1] The oldest of four children, she is a semiretired computer programmer who is a math whiz. She also loves antiques and quilting. But most significantly, she is a Washington Redskins football fan. Cheryl is easy to identify in her town between August and January. During these six months of the year, she sports a uniform—daily, she wears one of her 180 Washington Redskins football jerseys. At home, you'll find her walking around the house in her Redskins slippers. Her wardrobe is decidedly limited, but it suits her just fine. We wondered, on August 21, 1999, when she donated a kidney to a stranger, *was she wearing one of her jerseys in the operating room?* Even though the Baltimore Ravens were in town that day, playing her favorite team, it didn't derail her donation. She was ready to drop everything at a moment's notice. She's an altruist.

Cheryl had seen some television movies about organ donation in the past, but when she opened the newspaper and read an article about John, a man on dialysis for three years, she felt she was destined to be his donor. "God put the newspaper article in front of me."[2] She felt empathy for this man who was only six months older than herself (age fifty-three). An hour later, she picked up the telephone and called the operator, asking her to search for John's phone number. Getting her call, he was elated.

But the University of Maryland Medical Center was not as elated as John and Cheryl. In fact, when she called them to tell them the good news, they said they wouldn't consider her as a donor candidate because she wasn't John's friend or relative. That bit of information, while disappointing, fueled Cheryl to pursue the donation with even more passion. She met with John at a restaurant for a meal. Now, she could call herself a "friend." And now, she was acceptable to start the hospital's candidate assessment process. With the support of her husband and children, she completed the evaluation, assuring the donor team that her motivations were altruistic and that she had no intention of seeking monetary gain or fame for her donation. It helped that she had a prior history of altruism, namely, blood donation.

The day of surgery was a bit of a whirlwind for Cheryl. A defined surgery date had not been set because the hospital was waiting for the perfect arrangement of laboratory data for both John and Cheryl. She had a general idea of when the surgery would occur but not an exact day and time. She even notified her employer that if she didn't show up for work, the most logical place to find her would be in the operating room. Sure enough, Cheryl's husband was playing in a softball tournament, and she was out shopping with her family when the hospital called to notify her that they were ready for them. In fact, the hospital left eighteen voice mail messages on Cheryl's answering machine, desperately trying to contact her. Arriving home from shopping, she was met in her driveway by her daughter yelling, "Everybody is looking for you!"[3] She grabbed her prepacked overnight bag, drove to the athletic field, and picked up her husband, and off they went to the hospital.

Both the donation and the transplant surgeries went well. Two days after arriving home from the hospital, Cheryl was driving her car. But she had a strange feeling in her belly, and on occasion she saw something moving under her abdominal skin. During her routine follow-up visit at the doctor's office, she asked about it. The doctor explained how the contents of the pelvic cavity get shifted around during surgery, and he casually replied, "Oh, we forgot to tell you—that's your colon looking for a place to attach."[4] So even in the best of circumstances, donors should be prepared for the unexpected.

John's graft lasted nearly ten years before he died. During that time, Cheryl had a very close relationship with John and his wife, even helping to mediate their marital problems. She also was a significant presence at birthdays and holidays. She describes the donation experience as "wonderful"[5] and "rewarding"[6] and would repeat her decision to donate if she had the opportunity. For Cheryl, she has always felt that the donation from her to John was meant to happen and that it was God's plan for her life as well as John's.

Cheryl enjoys talking about her donation experience and continues her altruistic spirit in many ways, including volunteering with Meals on Wheels, a program that prepares and delivers food to those who are homebound. And you can't miss her car. It is the one with the bumper sticker that proudly proclaims, "Don't Take Your Organs to Heaven . . . Heaven Knows We Need Them Here!" In her case, she pleads for the organ procurement organization to "Salvage whatever they can use!"[7] after she passes away. She wants to transfer life to others as she leaves this world behind.

· 8 ·

Max: How Many
People Can I Help?

$\mathcal{S}$an Francisco and Clovis are two California cities that seem worlds apart even though the distance that separates them is only 163 miles. San Francisco is a large metropolitan city on the bay with towering skyscrapers, five-star hotels and restaurants, and its own professional baseball and football teams. Clovis sits in the agriculturally rich San Joaquin Valley at the foot of the Sierra Nevada mountain range and is known for its rodeo weekend every April. It has a country-western attitude that is laid back, compared to the bustling city life of San Francisco. And while Clovis does not have its own professional sports teams, it has produced several professional football players, including John Taylor (former wide receiver for the San Francisco 49ers), Daryle Lamonica (former quarterback for the Buffalo Bills and Oakland Raiders), and Zack Follett (linebacker for the Detroit Lions). Clovis also produced Good Samaritan kidney donor Max. His journey to kidney donation eventually took him to the University of California at San Francisco, where he gave the gift of life to a stranger in need.

Max was once a person in need. He had a troubled time during his youth and nearly died of a drug overdose. Our words can't begin to express his story, so we will let Max's own words speak directly to you:

> Quite some time ago in a hospital, doctor and nurses ran down a hallway to an emergency room. A life was about to be lost. Medical personnel made every attempt possible to revive and save this person, this person's life. These doctors and medical staff had left other duties to attend to one that may have been more critical than the one they were attending to at that time. After some time of not giving up, the life was restored and saved. That life that had been discouraged, depressed, and made some wrong choices which led to this emergency room visit. The doctors and nurses never gave up to save a life that was doomed. And that life was me.[1]

Max's trauma was an illicit drug overdose that nearly killed him. He was on leave from the military visiting his friends when he experimented with a drug that rendered him comatose. In fact, he was unaware of many of the details of the ordeal until his mother and hospital personnel explained matters to him. This event forever changed Max, and he has felt a "special calling"[2] in his life to help others. Max defines his special calling in the words of Albert Einstein: "Only a life lived for others is worth living."[3] And true to his heart, Max lives his life for others. As Max states,

> I realize now that there is a greater will for my life. . . . God made it possible for me to have another opportunity at life [and] I truly want to make the best of it! . . . I may have suffered through discouragement at times in my life, but we are not ultimately looked at by how many times we fall but by how many times we get up! I have chosen to press forward in life and make a difference! My Hope is that many others do also. . . . No matter what age we are, we can make a difference if we get up and press on forward. We will be like that tree planted by the water that sends out its roots by the stream. It will not fear when heat comes; its leaves are always green. It has no worries in a year of drought and never fails to bear fruit.[4]

The seventh of eleven children, Max was born to a housewife mother and a farm laborer father. He knows the concept of service very well. Thanks to his father, the community had fresh food on their tables. As a child, he wanted to be a fireman, but he eventually enlisted in the U.S. Air Force, serving for two years as an Italian translator in Sardinia, Italy. Now he is a department manager for the dairy, deli, and liquor units for one of the largest grocery store chains in California and Nevada. And it is at this grocery store where Max was challenged, literally, to be an organ donor.

Payday is always an important day for any employee, but this particular payday in 2009 was special. When Max looked at his pay stub, it looked different than usual. On the pay stub was a written challenge from his employer to consider participating as either a blood, a tissue, or an organ donor. He was already registered to donate his organs after death, but giving a kidney to someone as a living donor was something he had thought about before because he knew his nephew needed a kidney transplant.

Max had almost gotten to the point of donation once before. The thought would enter his mind, and he would drive to his local hospital and sit in the parking lot, waiting for more motivation to go in and ask for information about living donation. Until that remarkable summer payday, Max would drive off and return home. According to Max, God had been "tugging" at his heart, but he never followed through. The pay stub changed everything. With the challenge, he now had the stimulus to move forward. He volunteered to give a kidney to his nephew, but he already had five other living donor candidates pending. Then he heard about someone at his church who needed a kidney. This too was a dead end. Max, however, was not deterred. He pursued giving a kidney to a stranger and not just via a simple, straightforward donation; rather, he specifically chose chain donation.

At fifty years of age, Max began a chain of kidney donations that included twenty people across three states and saved ten lives. The person who received his kidney was twenty-seven-year-old Laura. She had been a vibrant college student until suddenly her body turned against her because of an autoimmune disease. Without a kidney transplant, she would die. Her brother, a willing donor, was not an immunological match. In stepped Max, and the donor shuffle began.

Max is also a special donor because he is Hispanic. In the United States, about 20 percent of the patients who received organ transplants in 2009 were Hispanic.[5] But very few Hispanics are living or deceased organ donors—only about 14 percent.[6] In 2009, there were 4,622 white and 933 Hispanic living donors in the United States.[7] Reasons for their low donation rates are likely complex. For example, it is known that Hispanic Americans have high rates of diabetes, obesity, high blood pressure, and heart disease. These conditions make one ineligible to participate as a living donor. They may also cause organ failure at the end of life, making donation after death impossible (even if the person had registered consent for donation). While we don't believe that language barriers are a factor because donation educational materials are generally published in a multitude of languages, there may be cultural influences that potentially impact donation decisions. The area is ripe for research.

Max's wife, Mary, has been very supportive of his volunteerism. When he told her that he wanted to be a donor and asked for her opinion about the idea, her first reaction was, "Wow, are you really sure you wanna do this?"[8] He assured her that that was his desire, and she supported him all the way. With a blended family, Max and his wife have five children, and they, too, were supportive. In a word, they are very proud of their father and amazed at the concept of Good Samaritan donation. For Max, "it actually means more to give to somebody you didn't know because you're really giving from the heart, you're not giving for any other reason but just to help somebody out."[9]

A man of faith, Max was never fearful about being a donor. He took things one step at a time and didn't worry. When his wife attended a few of the donor candidate screening appointments with him, she would ask questions, but Max always felt content and at peace. During the psychiatrist's evaluation, the clinician was amazed at the level of calm that Max expressed when talking about the concept of death. Donor candidates are always informed that there is a risk (very small) of death as a result of living donation. For example, the donor might have a stroke or cardiac arrest during or shortly after the surgery, or a hemorrhage could occur (a very remote risk). Max explained to the psychiatrist that he had no fears of dying and would live life to the fullest without the weight of fear on him. He explained that death is something that would be out of his control and that his faith in God gave him assurance that on death he would go to heaven, so he had no concerns. Throughout the process, his peace grew, and he never developed fears about participating as a donor. Even now, Max can't identify anything he is afraid of.

All but one of Max's children have left home now, but Max is not alone. He has his "surrogate daughter," the recipient of his kidney, Laura. When Max chose to be a Good Samaritan donor, he also chose to keep his identity private. He was content to complete his donor mission and return to his "regular" life, but when he learned that the recipient and her family were eager to meet him, he consented and feels that this encounter was important to them. They all remain very close, and Max supports their volunteer work, Dance for Donors,[10] an effort to increase donation awareness through music and dance. Max is also very active in his Protestant Evangelical church, leading Bible study groups, working with the elderly, and also conducting outreach ministry to those who are incarcerated. His employer also gave him a special award for his volunteerism. Max's donation to Laura made national news headlines,[11] and his story continues to be told as a witness of the power of donation and transplant. Max will live on through Laura and the others in the chain. He embodies altruism and has made giving to others a way of life.

· 9 ·

Jeff: Blind but with Clear Vision

It would be an understatement to say that Jeff knows a little bit about illness, loss, challenge, and overcoming. Jeff watched his father, trained as a chiropractor, endure sixty-three operations for mouth cancer complicated by excess radiation exposure. He is also the guardian and advocate for his severely cognitively disabled brother. Jeff lost his vision because of a lifelong progressive retinal disease, and he is now hard of hearing. His book, *Grit: A Family Memoir on Disability and Triumph*, is nearing completion. But lack of sight really seems to be the least noticeable attribute when we interviewed Jeff, as he is extremely articulate, intellectual, bold, creative, energetic, and passionate.[1] More prominent is the fact that at age sixty-one, he gave a kidney to a stranger.

As a child (the middle of three children), Jeff had many career dreams, including that of becoming a baseball player and an ice cream truck driver. But when his eyesight began failing at age five, his plans changed, and eventually his prosocial behaviors blossomed in full force. Jeff currently lives in Ohio and is a musician, songwriter, and disability advocate.[2] He has a collection of 250 instruments from around the world, twenty of which he plays. He has performed in forty-seven states in the United States, as well as internationally, and provided hundreds of concerts, free of charge, for hospice patients and their families who are moved to tears by the sentiments expressed in his lyrics. But it was his work in disability advocacy that led him to Good Samaritan organ donation. Specifically, he had been working for years with his business partner, Ward, to develop legislation supporting technology that provides accessible infrared signs with an audible voice for navigation assistance to those who can't see or read. Ward sent an email to his close circle of friends indicating that his daughter was in need of a kidney transplant. Her condition, kidney failure due to lupus, can cause weight gain, high blood pressure, dark urine (resulting from blood in the urine), and swelling around the eyes, legs, ankles, or fingers. Jeff responded, and a long, very long, process began. While Jeff was familiar with the burdens of kidney disease because he had known people who died before receiving a transplant, Jeff had no idea how difficult it was for a blind, older man to give a kidney to a stranger.

As you can imagine, Jeff is no wallflower. His lack of eyesight does not slow him down. He travels by train and plane, and he is very independent. But the process of living donor candidacy screening can be arduous, even for the sighted. The first transplant hospital he contacted declined to accept him as a donor, indicating that he was too old. They didn't even pursue a complete evaluation of him. (Did they not know about eighty-one-year-old Christine, who was a living kidney donor to her fifty-one-year-old son?[3]) The second hospital (in another state) accepted him but only after a very arduous process. Jeff's lack of sight requires that his travel plans be carefully formulated and include assistance along the way, so he had some tests performed at local facilities while others required travel out of state. In addition, he had to convince the donor team that just because he and the patient's father are business partners did not mean that Jeff was being paid to be an organ donor. Even though there were many hurdles, Jeff persevered because he felt that Good Samaritan organ donation was his "destiny."[4] As Jeff stated, "I could not *not* do it. It was given to me to do."[5] He didn't even care if he ever met the recipient: "It didn't matter."[6]

Two days before his surgery, Jeff attended an informational class about donation and transplantation at the hospital. There, he sang a song for the group, a song that he wrote for his recipient:[7]

> You spoke to me,
> I heard you in the night,
> You called my name.
> My soul was summoned,
> I woke and knew
> I'd never be the same.
> Selected,
> To accept donation's price,
> We are expected
> To relieve each other's strife;
> Time will fade
> All of the care-worn days,
> They'll pass as smoke.
> Come morning light
> With strength again
> You'll gladly lift your yoke.
> Selected
> To accept donation's price,
> We are expected

To save each others' life;
As I was meant to do,
I will say yes to you;
As I was meant to do,
I'll lay me down for you;

While these words likely touched the hearts of those who listened, for Jeff these words were full of meaning to him personally. A few weeks prior to surgery, he had received a phone call from his intended recipient. Rather than hearing a voice of excitement, Jeff heard a voice filled with tentativeness and anxiety. She expressed worries about her health, including the transplant process, medications, and organ rejection. Uncertain wonderings swirled: *What if Jeff donated and put his life on the line for her and her body rejected the organ? Did Jeff really want to donate? Was he going to change his mind and back out?* A surge of courage arose in Jeff, and he gently took charge of the conversation, consoling her and ministering to her fragility. Even his own fears about the donation surgery were swept away during the process.

So far, the recipient has done well with her transplant. Jeff has no regrets about donating and would repeat his decision to do so ("absolutely!"),[8] but his donation was not without medical consequences. During his hospitalization, he had an adverse reaction to the pain medication he received, causing severe hot, sticky itching. In addition, for some still unknown reason, he experienced chronic nausea for five months following his surgery. At the time of this writing, it has been about six months since his donation in 2009, and Jeff still occasionally battles this sickly "green" feeling. As Jeff is the type of person to "turn lemons into lemonade," his situation has motivated his desire to start a donor support group to help ensure that all living donors have access to peer support and other mechanisms for information and encouragement when they need it. He enjoys writing about his donation experience, and he is developing a living donor interview project with a major U.S. university hospital. When interviewed by National Public Radio about his donation experience, he never complained about his situation, and, in fact, he commented that the *recipient* would face more challenges than he because she has to take antirejection medications (immunosuppressants) for the rest of her life.[9]

It's hard to knock Jeff off his feet. He just plows forward. When he had pain and chronic nausea, he didn't let that stop him. Now he is advocating for the safety and welfare of living donors. Jeff says that "a great good resulted"[10] from his kidney donation. "Everything in my life, including my blindness and my brother's circumstance, taught me a great deal about the fact that the meaning of life is not to be found in the external."[11] He is certainly a prime example of someone who will not permit negative circumstances to affect either his quality of life or his ability to help others who are in need. He calls himself a "twenty-first-century Renaissance man,"[12] but we call him a Good Samaritan.

Jack: In Memory of
September 11

*J*ack is a charming and somewhat debonair former television newscaster and current director of communications and community relations for the largest suburb of Cleveland. Ohio may be a cold place to live most of the year, but we doubt that Jack ever notices the chilly temperatures and gray skies. He has a warm, upbeat personality. You would never know that under his professional business attire is a life-size color tattoo of a kidney emboldened on his lower back where his *real* kidney used to be. In 2007, Jack gave a kidney to a stranger.

The story started several years ago. Jack had witnessed his brother-in-law, Ken, endure dialysis for many years, but when his hand touched Ken's fistula, Jack became overwhelmed with empathy. A fistula is the surgical connection of a vein and an artery in the arm to allow rapid blood flow during dialysis. For Jack, there was something about feeling the blood whooshing underneath his fingertip. It opened the floodgates of emotions and thoughts about the burdens of dialysis that Ken had been enduring for all those years. Jack was determined to intervene.

Jack was tested to be a kidney donor to Ken, but he was not an immunological match. This, of course, did not stop Jack. Remember, this is a former television reporter who has the required tenacious streak in him. Jack enrolled in Ohio's Paired Donation Network.[1] This is an enterprise of nine Ohio hospitals that arrange living donor transplants using donors and patients who are immunologically incompatible at the time of their registration. These incompatible pairs are then shuffled (like a deck of cards) to create sets of compatible pairs. In 2010, the Paired Donation Network included more than eighty kidney transplant programs in twenty-three states that are organized in five regional consortia.

Jack was overjoyed to have found this program and thought the donation to Ken would be a slam dunk. As it turned out, there was no slam dunk at all. Jack and Ken waited a year and a half for a successful pair shuffle, but it never happened. The Paired Donation Network did not have the immunological match that Ken needed. But there *was* a match available, and it was right under Jack's nose—in fact, living in his house!

Lauren, twenty-four years old at the time, is Jack's daughter. Lauren volunteered to donate and was a match. Jack and his wife, understandably, were concerned for their daughter as any parent would be. Lauren is a young, single mother to a five-year-old child. But Lauren persisted, and so did Jack. He was not going to stop the process he had started with the Paired Donation Network. Lauren donated to Ken, and Jack donated to a stranger to whom he matched.[2] All this made for a very eventful experience for Jack's wife because the surgeries involved having her three closest relatives all in operating rooms at the same time (her spouse, her daughter, and her brother). Now that requires emotional stamina!

Looking back, Jack recalls all that his wife was going through and thinks that maybe there were times when he was a bit tunnel visioned with his efforts to press forward with donating. Now he realizes donation as a family affair that must regularly reflect on the concerns and needs of all the relatives who are impacted. Jack and his wife have been married for more than thirty years. He knows that communication is important to a successful relationship but admits that he could have been a better communicator at times during the donation evaluation process. Even if a spouse or child is supportive of another's desire to donate, they still might have fears, anxiety, and questions that need answering. Planning for the event and aftercare is a team effort of the whole family, not just the intending donor.

Through the paired donation experience, Jack was able to help get two people off dialysis: his brother-in-law and a stranger. The latter young man had been enduring several years of home peritoneal dialysis, tethered to a machine in the evenings after arriving home from work. Jack describes the donation as a euphoric and rewarding event. He has no regrets about donating and would repeat his decision to do so if given the opportunity. According to Jack, "The result for the donors and recipients was nothing but positive. You can't ask for more than that."[3] And Jack's own words are the best explanation for his altruism:

> In my heart I wanted to make a difference. I feel that's why I was put on earth to make a difference in making life better for an individual or group of individuals. I'm always concerned about people who have less than I have, and I think we have a responsibility to take care of one another. I

do believe that there's a reason why we're here, and that's to help those in need. I am not a hero. I am no better than anyone else. I call myself a helper. . . . I consider my contribution to society as being one of the most powerful things that a person can do.[4]

Like nearly all the Good Samaritan donors we interviewed, Jack had no fears about the surgery. "If it was meant to happen it was going to happen. . . . If it wasn't meant to happen it wasn't going to happen."[5] Even on the day of surgery, as he was being wheeled into the operating room, Jack was laughing and joking. "I really considered it to be more or less out of my hands and in the hands of a higher being."[6] Indeed, his religious upbringing (Catholic) helped guide him to volunteer activities and helped him feel at peace with the decision to donate. The youngest of three, his parents were role models for him and taught him to help others and "do the right thing."[7] For Jack, donation was the "right" thing to do.

Jack is fifty-seven years old, but he looks much younger, and he credits this to his daily workout routine. In addition, his service work continues. He is a mentor to other living donors, helping them understand the donation process. This mentoring and encouragement can also be helpful during the recovery period, when donors might be experiencing pain or other surgical side effects. Overall, service runs in the family for Jack. When he was a child growing up, he wanted to be a firefighter like his dad. His daughter, Lauren, is a firefighter-paramedic. Jack has served the community as a journalist and continues to serve by way of vocal presence supporting organ donation. He'd like to be a liver lobe donor, but the procedure is too risky for him. Instead, both he and his wife participate in platelet donation every two weeks. "I've always gravitated toward volunteering and helping out."[8]

When Jack was given a choice of dates for his donation, he chose September 11. He wanted something good to happen on that date so that every year, when most of us remember the horror of September 11,[9] he remembers that he saved a life. When he dies, Jack looks forward to being an organ donor again because he is registered as a deceased donor. "When I die someone's going to hit the lottery because my organs are going everywhere!"[10]

III

SERVING OTHERS
AND GIVING BACK

Trends among Good Samaritans

My life feels so much better when I do what I can for other people.

—Nicole, Good Samaritan kidney donor[1]

SERVING OTHERS

*W*hile interviewing our twenty-two Good Samaritan donors, we observed two prominent themes: serving others and giving back to society. It is no coincidence that we can also extract these two concepts from the principle of altruism. This is because "others" and "society" relate to the concept of "neighbors," and serving and giving back are behaviors that benefit our neighbors. Observing these themes, we took a closer look and explored the occupations (and childhood aspirations) of our twenty-two donors as well as their personal history of volunteerism.

Good Samaritan organ donors transform lives through their donation, but many also do so by way of the fact that they have service-oriented occupations. Specifically, service-oriented occupations transform others when people learn from teachers, are cared for by doctors and nurses, are protected and rescued by police and firefighters, are advocated for by attorneys, and are spruced up by hairdressers. Service-oriented occupations are not focused on producing a product; rather, they are concerned with imparting change—improving or helping something, someone, or a situation. Of our twenty-two donors, sixteen (73 percent) were employed in service-oriented jobs at the time of their donation, and one was on active duty in the military (voluntary enlistment). Three of sixteen (19 percent) were employed in the health care sector (nurse midwife, psychologist, or occupational therapist), and another plans on becoming a nurse. In fact, of the nineteen donors who had a concrete answer to the question, "When you were a child, what did you want to be when you grew up?," fourteen (74 percent) responded with a service-oriented occupation (half indicating either "social worker" or a health care profession and nearly 30 percent indicating a protective role such as fireman, policeman, or park ranger).

With 74 percent of our Good Samaritan donors desiring a service-oriented occupation as a child, we wondered if this might have anything to do with their role models. To explore this concept, we identified the occupations of the parents of each of our twenty-two donors. Most mothers were "housewives" (twelve of twenty-two), but of those who worked outside the home, two-thirds were employed in the service sector as health care workers or teachers. With regard to the donors' fathers, nine of twenty-two (41 percent) were employed in the service sector (three health care workers and one social worker). Some service-oriented occupations have the concept of volunteerism innately built in, such as health care and law. Doctors and attorneys, for example, are customarily expected to provide some pro bono services. Firefighters don't invoice those rescued for their services (though this is changing in some U.S. municipalities).

Could it be that witnessing and experiencing the helping-oriented professions leads to civic attitudes and behaviors such as volunteering? Could such prosocial attitudes and behaviors be groomed from an early age? Psychologist David Rosenhan thinks so. His research concluded that there is a significant relationship between parental modeling of altruistic behavior and altruistic behaviors by their adult children.[2] Four of our donors also believe this to be true, as they offered commentary that identified their upbringing and relatives as contributing to their volunteerism.

Eight of our twenty-two donors (36 percent) were involved in community volunteer activities prior to and/or after organ donation. These activities include Rotary, working with dying patients in hospitals and nursing homes, Boy Scouts of America, community education, and pastoral care for those who are incarcerated. Volunteer activities, combined with service sector occupations, seemed the tip of the prosocial behavior iceberg for many of our Good Samaritan donors. This is because as we explored further, there were even *more* altruistic-spirited activities that were part of their lives.

Military service is another example of volunteerism. In the United States, for example, while all males ages eighteen to twenty-five are required by law to register with the Selective Service for potential military drafting, current military service (active duty and reserves) is based on volunteerism. In fact, individuals lose many of their civilian rights when they enlist, so their dedication and sense of duty is noteworthy. Service in the military is an extreme form of volunteerism because individuals essentially devote themselves to their government and community and potentially put themselves at risk of bodily harm. In some ways, this is similar to Good Samaritan organ donation: volunteering for the benefit of unidentified recipients and exposure to personal risk (including the risk of death and morbidity) so that the recipient can benefit. Interviewing our twenty-two donors, we identified seven (32 percent) with a military history. Two of seven are women. Specifically, one donor is an active member of the air force, and six others have served in various branches of the military, including Special Forces (paracommando rescuing captured soldiers). Many of their parents also had a military history (eleven of twenty-two fathers). Parental military service, a prosocial behavior (though some enlistments were likely via a mandatory draft rather than volunteerism), may have been another area of modeling that prompted prosocial behavior in their offspring.

Returning to the medical context, we found that most of our twenty-two Good Samaritan organ donors pursued blood or marrow donation prior to their organ donation. Specifically, nineteen of twenty-two (86 percent) had been blood donors, and five of twenty-two (23 percent) had registered to be bone marrow donors. Prior to their Good Samaritan organ donation, one had performed bone marrow donation, and another had given a kidney to a relative. Our findings are very similar to what has been reported in the medical literature. In two studies researching the characteristics of Good Samaritan kidney donors, both found a significant portion had participated as blood or marrow donors prior to donation.[3] In their study of Good Samaritan liver donors, Reichman et al. found that ten of twelve (83 percent) donors had donated blood or were registered as potential bone marrow donors prior to their organ donation.[4] Considering that blood and marrow donations are also altruistic, there seems to be a pattern of prosocial behavior by Good Samaritan organ donors, and this pattern spans both medical and nonmedical arenas. Because only five of twenty-two of our donors expressed any fear about their donation procedure, organ donation can be viewed as a logical next step (from blood or marrow donation). Indeed, several donors made comments to this effect when they stated their motivations for donating. With a history of bone marrow donation, Karen remarked, "What else can I do? . . . if I wait any longer I might not be able to give anything."[5]

GIVING BACK

The concept of "giving back" can be viewed as serving others with or without the expectation of a return (reciprocity). Several of our twenty-two donors told us stories of their contented lives and how their "fortunate" life situation led them to desire to give back in a significant way. While many of our donors were not wealthy (yearly family income less than $75,000), about half reported annual incomes in excess of $100,000 at the time of their donation. Some of these individuals could possibly have chosen to make monetary donations to transplant-affiliated charities, for example, but none did; instead, they chose organ donation as their way of giving back. *Why an organ and not money?*

For our donors, it seems that logic prevailed. They knew that money was not what patients in organ failure need; rather, they need a new organ. As Nicole so aptly put it, "Why are there so many people walking around with two perfectly health kidneys when they only need one?"[6] Fred, also a kidney donor, felt the same way: "There's gotta be somebody that needs one [of mine]."[7] Josie was in the situation of wanting to donate to her spouse, but since she was not a compatible blood type, she gave a kidney to a stranger who needed one, and someone else gave a kidney to her husband (as part of a chain). Again, money was not the primary need for these patients; rather, it was the organ.

The contented life spoken about by donors was an all-encompassing concept referring to financial soundness, personal happiness and health, and career success. Not only did this give them the freedom and ability to donate, but it gave several the sense that they had a duty to give back because they had so much (compared to others). As Maureen stated, "When you're among the lucky people, then, you know, more will be expected of you."[8] Jack, a kidney donor in Ohio told us, "It's just been a very lucky life that I've had. I'm always concerned about people who have less than I have, and I think we have a responsibility to take care of one another."[9] Deborah told us, "You have to give back. I have been very lucky in my life."[10] Max, a kidney donor stated, "God has blessed me with good health to be able to help somebody else."[11] Even more interesting is the fact that these donors expressed no fears about donating—perhaps they felt that their providence would continue in terms of experiencing no surgical complications. One developed a minor a postoperative bladder infection easily treated with antibiotics. Another developed an incisional hernia that required surgical repair and several months off work to recover. Even so, none have any regrets about donating.

Another element of "giving back" is the belief in the concept of a "higher good."[12] Indeed, for six of twenty-one of our donors (one was lost to follow-up), this was very important as indicated by their score on the Volunteer Motivation Inventory.[13] Four of twenty-one donors ranked this as the primary motivator for volunteering, and two more gave it a tie ranking with the motivation of helping others ("values"). The creators of the Volunteer Motivation Inventory assign the term "reciprocity" to motivations based on the concept of a higher good because they believe that these individuals view their volunteer activities as being part of an "equal exchange" that will bring about good things in the future.

Notice that this giving back and future "good things" is not an explicit attempt to gain favor or earn a reward. These donors aren't donating an organ now because they might need one in the future if they get sick (however, they will get preference in receiving a deceased organ donation if they subsequently suffer organ failure).[14] Our Good Samaritans who subscribe to reciprocity as a motivator gave an organ because it is a method of giving back to the community, delivering good to the community from their personal, bountiful pool of providence. As Garrett, a kidney donor, stated, "We have to get along and take care of each other when we can."[15] Similar thoughts were conveyed by Cynthia, also a kidney donor: "What I can I will do."[16] Both donors scored reciprocity as their primary motivator on the Volunteer Motivation Inventory.

What we identified in our donors has also been thoroughly studied by psychologists and termed a norm of generalized reciprocity.[17] Critical to this behavior is the fact that the giver does not need the receiver's help. In addition, the giver gives without strings attached—there is not an expectation from the giver that the recipient will do anything in return or react in a certain way. Similarly, altruists live to give, not to receive. They don't give with a list of preconditions attached. We confirmed these concepts when interviewing our Good Samaritan donors. Specifically, most donors commented that they had no desire to choose who received their organ. Dave and Cheryl, however, were unique exceptions. As discussed earlier, Dave believes that he was chosen by God to give to a specific teenager whom he saw on television in need of a lung transplant and did not want to deviate from God's plan.[18] Dave had no desire to meet the boy, only to be his donor. Cheryl told a similar story; namely, she believes that it was God's plan for her to give to the man she read about in the newspaper, although she had no desire to know him.[19] In these two situations, both donors feel that they did not choose their organ recipients but rather that God chose them. Similarly, only one donor indicated that meeting the recipient was a critical to the donation experience. This kidney donor wanted to personally see the benefit that the patient received in order to make the donation experience "more real."[20] Another donor admitted that after donating, she developed an intense curiosity about her organ recipient and has been trying to determine his or her identity using the Internet.[21]

MAXIMIZING THE GOOD

Ethicists seek to maximize good while minimizing harm. Not only do altruists want to do good for others, but the concept of maximizing the good appears as well. We first saw this when donors made the medical leap from blood and marrow donation to solid organ donation. While all three are potentially lifesaving, organs are much scarcer than blood or marrow, and thus the donation is so precious. Several of our donors did not stop at the straightforward concept of organ donation; rather, they took another leap forward to paired donation (Jack) and chain donation (Max, Cynthia, and Josie). As mentioned, in paired donation, the donor's original intent is to give an organ to a specific individual (usually a spouse, relative, or friend) but is blood type incompatible, so the incompatible pair is matched up with another incompatible pair and then shuffled to make two compatible pairs, with two donors each giving to two strangers. In this way, one transplant becomes two. We consider the donations that occur amid paired donation a form of Good Samaritan donation because the recipients are strangers. Sometimes, these pairs never meet.

Chain donation works like a cascade of falling dominoes and creates a series of transplants. A Good Samaritan donor (the first domino in the cascade) starts the chain of transplants that occurs between pairs that were once incompatible and ends with either a donation to someone who was waiting for a deceased donor organ (didn't originally have a living donor option) or a bridge donor who can start a new chain of donations to people who have incompatible live donor matches. Chain donation allows the Good Samaritan donor to help many patients get their needed transplants by starting the transplant cascade. For kidney donor Max, this was exactly his intent. He was given information about paired donation but specifically opted for chain donation so that he could "help more people."[22] To date, the longest chain consists of twenty-one transplants.[23]

A third (and controversial) method of maximizing benefit was also of interest to some of our Good Samaritan donors: multiple organ donation. In a subsequent chapter, we will present the story of Deborah, who was an organ donor on two separate occasions. The first time, she gave a kidney to her father. Next, she gave a liver lobe to a child whose photo she saw on a flyer. These types of donations are extremely rare. Removing an organ from a healthy person on one occasion is risky enough for most surgeons, so the thought of doing it twice is generally out of the question. Nonetheless, at least four of our Good Samaritan donors have expressed interest in donating another organ, and three have undergone screening but were ruled out for medical reasons (new onset diabetes, potential blood coagulation disorder, or being at high risk for complications). We view multiple donations as a concept that requires deep exploration by multidisciplinary donor teams. Specifically, while altruism is a good, there must be assurance that some other, harmful mechanism is not in play. For example, there are known cases of clinically unneeded amputations that patients have demanded for their own psychological "benefit."[24] A case of a Good Samaritan kidney donor desiring to continue to donate to the point of suicide has also been reported.[25] Organ donor advocacy requires that individuals be protected from harm and not be allowed to donate when it is not in their best interest. This is why the work of transplant ethicists is vital to fostering donor safety as well as the integrity of transplant as a profession.

· *12* ·

Deborah: Twice a Donor!

*D*eborah is a bookkeeper by occupation, but she is also an expert at living donation. *Do you want to know what it is like to donate a kidney?* Deborah can tell you all about it as she gave one of hers to her father. *Do you want to know the details of liver donation?* Deborah knows about that too. She donated a liver segment to a child, someone who was a stranger to her. She will tell you that liver donation is actually a lot like childbirth in terms of the pain and also because, after all the pain is over, you are "blessed"[1] by the outcome.

There are some people who go through life always seeing the positive. It doesn't matter what the situation is: the glass is always half full. Deborah laughs easily and gets full enjoyment out of every experience. She is a natural caretaker. When her father needed a kidney transplant, she and her siblings went to be tested. All were perfect immunological matches, but Deborah, the eldest, felt that it was her responsibility to make sure her younger siblings did not put themselves at risk (even though the risks of living kidney donation are minimal). As Deborah told us, she overruled them all. In addition, looking back, she describes the steps of her journey as all lining up perfectly, as if they were meant to be.

Deborah's journey as a Good Samaritan liver donor started when she was working on a cancer fund-raiser. Specifically, she was handing out flyers for a sixty-mile fund-raising walk. She happened to give a flyer to a friend who was fund-raising for another endeavor, and soon after, this friend faxed her a flyer for his quest. On the flyer was the photo of a three-year-old Hispanic boy in need of a liver transplant. Deborah placed the flyer in her desk drawer at work, and every time she opened the drawer, she saw the child's face looking back at her. "He was just so cute!"[2] If Deborah has a weakness, it's a child in need. Seeing him look at her all day long was enough to move her to call the number on the flyer and request a donor candidacy evaluation.

Having been through the kidney donation experience, she knew there would be testing and a series of interviews involved, but she underestimated the extent of the screening process for liver donation. At the Cleveland Clinic in Ohio, one of the most experienced transplant centers in the world, they put her through a rigorous assessment process. This was not only because liver donation is a much more complex surgery than kidney donation (and with more risks), but also because she had already had four trips to the operating room in the past (three childbirths and the kidney donation). Multiorgan donors are exceedingly rare, and the hospital had to be assured that Deborah was a safe surgical candidate. They also had to be assured that she was psychologically healthy and possessed an altruistic motivation. There are some psychological pathologies that involve people seeking to give away or remove their body parts for reasons that have *nothing* to do with altruism (e.g., body integrity identity disorder[3]). Donations from these individuals are ethically inappropriate. While Deborah knew that her motivations were pure, the hospital needed assurance. She was interviewed by a social worker, a psychiatrist, and a clinical ethicist. Passing all these assessments, as well as the medical and surgical evaluations, Deborah was approved to donate.

Appropriately, Deborah was reflective as to how her family felt about her desire to donate another organ. Her husband is a federal air marshal and formerly spent time in Iraq and Afghanistan doing Special Forces operations for the U.S. Army. Even though he understands the concept of risk very well, initially he wasn't excited about the idea of a second donation. Deborah then reminded him about all the times he volunteered for high-risk activities and suggested he stop—he then understood the irony, laughed at the role reversal, and supported Deborah all the way. Her twenty-six-year-old daughter, as well as her sister, also eventually voiced their support after initially expressing strong concerns against her donation.

In an unusual occurrence, Deborah met the child and his family (parents and grandmother) prior to surgery. The family wanted to meet her and thank her in advance for her generosity. With her consent, the family arranged for a meeting at the food court of a nearby shopping mall. Deborah never had any plans to meet the recipient or his family, but she did not want to deprive them of this opportunity. In the setting of a slight language barrier (the family's primary language is Spanish), the look in their eyes said it all. They were so grateful for the gift about to be received.

In 2009, Deborah gave the gift of life. She experienced a six-week recovery from surgery but had no complications other than pain. She describes the healing process as slow but indicates that she has "no limitations"[4] and gives accolades to her living donor coordinator, Peggy, for being extremely helpful with information and support throughout the entire process. "She was amazing . . . my buddy . . . every step of the way."[5]

Deborah follows the progress of both her organ recipients. Her father is doing well, but the child has developed a complication: non-Hodgkin's lymphoma (a cancer originating in white blood cells in the lymphatic system). At times, he is readmitted to the hospital for care. This setback does not upset Deborah. She has no regrets about donating and would repeat her decision to do so if given the opportunity. She has also thought about pursuing living lung donation as well as bone marrow donation.

Even though she is very satisfied with her donation experience, she does not actively promote living donation because she believes that it is a very personal experience involving risk. In fact, compared to other Good Samaritan donors we interviewed, Deborah's story is silent on the Internet. There are no articles, blogs, Web pages, or other online literature detailing her donation. As she told us, "Everybody has to completely come to that choice on their own."[6] She gave the gift not only because she was moved by empathy when seeing the photo of the ill child but also because she believes that she has had a very "lucky"[7] life and that because of her good fortune she has an obligation "to give back."[8] Her life has not changed other than feeling that she has given someone the "perfect"[9] gift—just what a little boy needed.

· *13* ·

Missy: I Can Give Life

*W*ith her long dark hair and bangs, you'd never believe Missy is old enough to have been a practicing psychologist for more than twenty-five years. But, in fact, she is almost sixty. She has a rich, easy laugh and a great sense of humor, which, given her chosen profession, is a great gift both to herself and to her clients. And while you might think of a Quaker as a quiet, unassuming person, Missy has made a very bold statement: she gave a kidney to a stranger.[1]

The younger of two children, maybe she learned about being bold from her father, a lieutenant general in the U.S. Marine Corps. She certainly had focus about her life at an early age. By ninth grade, she knew she wanted to be a psychologist, and she followed her dream. She spent the first portion of her career in San Diego teaching psychotherapy at the graduate level. Eventually, she became a specialist in substance abuse (she is a recovering alcoholic herself) and pain management for chronic illness. Working with clients on changing thinking and behavior, talk therapy is only one of her tools. She uses different techniques in her practice, including self-hypnosis for cancer patients and others suffering from debilitating diseases in order to deal with the burdensome side effects of medication and radiation therapy.

Missy never had any personal connection to donation or transplant and didn't have any friends or family on dialysis. One day in 2006, while she was aboard an airplane, she began reading a book about compassion and altruism.[2] She hoped to use material from the book to prepare a lecture for her psychology students. But two chapters of the book, both focused on living donation, moved her deeply, and she decided to become a kidney organ donor at her alma mater, the University of North Carolina at Chapel Hill.

Missy's donation was not uneventful. The screening process took many months and had its stops and starts because of various clinical findings that appeared during her testing. Eventually, she was cleared to donate, but during the surgery there was a complication—her spleen was nicked with a surgical tool during the laparoscopic procedure, and she began to hemorrhage a large quantity of blood. The surgical team had to quickly intervene and convert the procedure to an "open" technique using a large abdominal incision. Her spleen was removed, and she received a large transfusion of blood that saved her life. Her recovery period was painful and prolonged because of this complication, but Missy was able to use self-hypnosis as a helpful intervention. Missy is the only one of our twenty-two donors to have a life-threatening event as a result of living donation, but she indicates that she was aware of the risk and has no regrets about her decision. In fact, she feels that, overall, she has "better health,"[3] and she lost weight after donating.

Throughout the process, Missy had the support of her boyfriend, even though he was anxious. Missy, too, was not without fear. She worried about possible complications or even death, but she wanted to donate. When the testing process became lengthy, laborious, and inconvenient, Missy held steadfast, motivated by the words of the venipuncture technicians.[4] Serendipitously, one of the technicians who had drawn her blood the day before was the mother of the intended recipient. And the technician who was sampling her blood the following day wanted to be the donor but was unable to do so. Missy was able to comfort this technician—to help alleviate her feelings of sadness and guilt. In addition, the experience made Missy suddenly aware of how donation decisions affect people and can cause others to become very reflective and awed by the goodness of prosocial acts.

Looking back on her experience, Missy put her skills as a psychologist to work when she prepared an educational pamphlet for her transplant hospital.[5] Because on several occasions she came very close to *not* donating (because of test results during her clinical evaluation), she became keenly aware of the emotional stress this caused her, and she wanted to avert this stress in others. Portions of the pamphlet text are presented below with permission:

> As you take each step along the way, something may stop the process— you're not the match you had hoped for, there's an unexpected health risk, a loved one can't tolerate the thought of your donation, or there is so much on your plate emotionally that it would be a mental risk for you to undergo a procedure that asks so much of you. However you come to the point of realizing that you can't donate as you had hoped, you will likely experience many confusing feelings. You might experience a mixture of relief, guilt, sadness, anger, disappointment or emptiness—all at once, or you might experience one feeling at one moment and shift to another the next and then back again. On top of that, there may be intense loneliness as those around you have their own feelings and may not truly understand what you are experiencing. Please know that all of these confusing, changing feelings are normal, and shared by others who have been on a similar journey to yours.

One particularly difficult feeling is guilt, which can take the form of "survivor guilt," which sounds like "Why do I get to keep all my organs when someone who needs one is still in trouble?" Or the guilt of simply not being able to provide what you know someone else needs. That feeling may get even bigger if you notice the very understandable feeling of some relief in not being able to donate. That relief is part of being human—it doesn't mean you care any less. It doesn't mean you're selfish. It's the natural reaction to not having to go through a difficult, demanding experience.

Another tough one is the feeling of being inadequate or a failure—that there's something about you that isn't good enough to donate. That can be a very subtle feeling of feeling badly about yourself or your body, of not measuring up in some way. If you have had any areas of self-doubt in your life as most people have, the determination that you can't be a donor can heighten old feelings of failure. You take a hit emotionally.

No matter what the reason, and whether you feel guilt, relief or a sense of failure, the decision that you can't donate always involves loss. If you've been invested in the process for a while, the loss is even bigger—you've been through medical testing . . . and testing . . . and testing . . . and talking to many, many people about the possibility of donation. All of that stops. The wish, the hope, the investment of time and energy, the imagination of the future—all of that may change in an instant and you're left with emptiness. The disappointment and grief may be surprising, even if you thought you were prepared for the possibility that it might not happen. That's what grief is—the mind's way of trying to come to terms with loss, and it might go on for a while. This is a time when it might be useful to talk to someone about your experience about normal but difficult feelings. You might consider talking to a counselor connected to a transplant program or in your community. If your feelings cause you questions or conflict with your faith, you may want to talk to your pastor or to contact pastoral care at the hospital. Talking to someone uninvolved in this process can be very helpful.

No matter the reason for not being able to donate, it's important to realize that your real consideration of donating is powerful and important all in its own right. The efforts and investment you've made, for however long the journey has been—short or long—are not wasted. They have had enormous impact in ways you may not even realize.

Missy feels fortunate to have been able to donate. As she told us, "If you know you can, how can you not? I live pretty close to my value system, believing pretty strongly about needing to contribute in the world."[6] Even though she never met the man who received her organ and knows nothing about him, this has not dampened her experience. "I can't give birth, but I can give life."[7]

IV

THE GIFT OF GIVING

· *14* ·

Saints or Normal Folk?

$\mathscr{B}$y now, I think we have adequately dispelled the myth that Good Samaritan organ donors are "crazy." But other questions remain: Are they "super saints" or just "normal" members of the community? Do Good Samaritan organ donors have ultra-virtuous tendencies that exceed "usual and customary" helping behavior (whatever that is)? Could anyone be a Good Samaritan or just special people? Consider for a moment the donation story of Rabbi Ephraim Simon, a husband as well as a father to nine young children, aged two to fourteen, in New Jersey.[1] He was motivated to donate a kidney to a stranger after receiving a mass-mailed email from a woman who was trying to find a kidney donor for a child in need. While he was not a match for the child, he was still motivated to donate, believing it would be a lifesaving gift from him, his wife, and his children to the recipient. He underwent testing for several potential recipients (all strangers) and was finally matched to a man who was the father of ten children. The rabbi's view is that he used his own excellent health to help someone else. Not only is the rabbi a parent to his nine children, but one of *his* kidneys allowed the patient to continue *his* parental role to ten children.

Does John Feal have extraordinary goodness, or is he just regular folk?[2] John, a former army soldier, was among the first to arrive on the scene in New York City on September 11, 2001, after the Twin Towers were attacked by terrorists. He moved debris to help enable the rescue and recovery of victims. John lost a foot during this heroic volunteer work (it was amputated after being crushed by a beam) and suffered from exposure to toxic compounds. Nonetheless, his beneficent acts and volunteerism continued. He donated a kidney to a stranger in 2007 and also created the FealGoodFoundation, an organization dedicated to advocacy, education, and relief efforts for 9/11 volunteer workers with resultant health problems.[3] John replied to an email from a stranger who was seeking a kidney transplant. The stranger, a volunteer firefighter who had also worked at the 9/11 site, had asked John if he would spread the word about his need for a kidney, but John said there was no need for that, as he would give him one of *his* kidneys. While he was not a match to the stranger, he entered a paired donation,[4] and two incompatible pairs were shuffled to make two compatible pairs ("matches"). John hopes to spread the word about the need for organ transplants among 9/11 rescue workers, including those who need lung transplants as a result of exposure to toxic dust.

Joe Rosner is another Good Samaritan. Raised in a gang-infested area of Chicago, he witnessed the brutality and pain of violence. When his best friend was sexually attacked, Joe became impassioned to help defend the vulnerable. Joe became an expert on safety and self-defense and authored a book, *Street Smarts and Self-Defense for Children: A Parent's Guide*.[5] He also formed a company, Best Defense, which teaches children, health care workers, real estate agents, and the community how to protect themselves from violence, bullying, and abuse.[6] But Joe's aid to the vulnerable did not stop there. He volunteered with the Red Cross during times of flooding, and in 2006 he donated a kidney to a stranger in New York. According to his wife, organ donation was the path he was meant to be on, and she was not going to steer him away from it.[7] *Are good deeds his gift?*

CARING THINKING

Could anyone be a Good Samaritan or just special people? Some people are "gifted" in areas such as music, sports, art, or math. *Do Good Samaritans have the gift of extraordinary giving?* People with psychiatric disorders that render them unable to experience empathy seem unable to be Good Samaritans. Even lacking a psychiatric diagnosis, it would seem that those who are unable to look beyond their own needs to respond to the needs of others are incapable of Good Samaritan behavior. This said, it is likely that most people *do* have the functional capacity to be Good Samaritans in some format. While we have presented the stories of people who might appear ready to be canonized, it seems that Good Samaritan organ donors are the people you would meet during your week: the barista at your favorite café,[8] the janitor at your church or office,[9] or the plumber who repairs your broken faucet.[10] They all have the same things in common: they are other-oriented, empathetic, helpful people. Good Samaritans are the people who rise to the occasion—their desire to help does not compete with and lose out to other goals, such as career or financial success;

rather, it's all compatible. They haven't taken vows of poverty to then live in their cars so that others can live in houses. They have life pursuits and goals like most people, but they also allow prominent space for giving, and they don't allow self-serving goals (even if present) to conquer or diminish their norm of helpfulness. They might take a break from a "helping" pursuit, but they won't be derailed from their commitment to it.

Consider Zachary Sutton.[11] At twenty-eight years old, he decided to take a short break from his schoolwork. He was studying to be a physician's assistant at the Medical University of South Carolina. As an adult, he had witnessed the suffering of his grandfather with end-stage kidney disease and dialysis. Earlier in his life, as a child, he had observed a family donate their son's organs when he was killed in a car accident. Zachary committed himself to be a Good Samaritan organ donor to someone he never met. While Zachary is white, the recipient of his perfectly matched kidney, Michael Cheeks, is black. Race is irrelevant when it comes to organ matching. Michael had been waiting fifteen years for a kidney when Zachary came along. Sutton insists he is a "normal guy, not a saint."[12]

Matt Jones has been called an "angel."[13] In 2007, this twenty-eight-year-old father of four gave a kidney to a stranger. He had to take a break from his college classes and full-time work at his car rental job to do it, but he was more than happy to. He equated kidney donation to dropping coins in the Salvation Army red kettle during the holidays. He had watched a television program about donation and learned that humans only need one healthy kidney to live a normal life. As he stated, "So if you've got something a little extra that you don't need and someone else could use it to live a decent life, I believe you should share it."[14]

And then there is "Pillar of the Community," Kay Wolff.[15] A retired elementary school principal, Kay became a Good Samaritan kidney donor at the age of seventy-two.[16] One might think she should be content in her retirement—sit back and relax or maybe knit and play a little bingo or golf. Not Kay: she is a giver. In the past, she had wanted to give a kidney to friends who needed it, but she wasn't a match. Having seen the suffering of those on dialysis, she was not deterred and pursued living donation to a stranger. Even being told she was "too old" by one transplant center did not derail her donation desire. She contacted another center that was willing to thoroughly evaluate her. In 2010, Kay gave a kidney to a sixty-three-year-old woman who had been on dialysis for six years. They met for the first time on the day of surgery when they walked into the hospital elevator simultaneously. Kay has a long history of helping, including establishing twenty acres of hiking trails within the Fred Wolff Bear Creek Nature Preserve in California as well as being a member of the Community Emergency Response Team (CERT).

CERT members respond during disasters and are trained to manage utilities and put out small fires; assist victims with breathing, control bleeding, and treat for shock; provide basic medical aid; and search for and rescue victims safely.

All these Good Samaritan donors appear to have something in common: caring thinking. What is fascinating about "caring thinking" is that it emerges from the field of gifted education (practices, procedures, and theories used in the education of children who have been identified as gifted or talented). In fact, we had put forth the thought question, *Do Good Samaritans have the gift of extraordinary giving?* The "normal" world would argue that giving a vital organ to a stranger is "crazy," but for a "gifted" person, this could be *their* norm. For "normal folk" the expectation would be to keep one's own body parts for one's own physical function or, at most, to donate to a friend or relative in need. But Good Samaritans defy this "normal" expectation. Along these lines, psychologist Martha Morelock has stated,

> If development is perceived as a life-long process, giftedness can then be understood as producing atypical development throughout the lifespan in terms of awareness, perceptions, emotional responses, and life experiences. This places the gifted individual developmentally out of sync both internally, in relation to the different aspects of development, and externally, in relation to cultural expectations.[17]

According to educational theorist Jan Brunt, caring thinking ("the new intelligence") is thinking that stems from the heart and reflects one's personal values.[18] She argues that the behavior of caring thinkers is motivated by "intense social and moral conscience" and that it has four components: valuational thinking, affective thinking, active thinking, and normative thinking.[19] Valuational thinking "underpins the establishment of ethical principles."[20] It involves appreciating things not for their monetary worth but, rather, for their other appeals (sensory, visual, emotional, and personal). Affective thinking is the experience of an emotional and cognitive response to injustice. Caring thinkers have a strong sense of justice and are emotionally upset when encountering injustice. They are also sensitive to the feelings of others and are very empathetic. They have strong notions about "right and wrong."

The active thinking element of caring thinking finds the individual taking steps to solve problems (e.g., responding to relieve suffering). This is where altruistic motivations become altruistic behaviors. Merging empathetic reactions with the desire for justice, one can see how altruistic behaviors such as advocacy and volunteerism emerge from caring thinkers. The sincerity and commitment of the caring thinker blossom into other-oriented behavior. The normative thinking element of caring thinking calls on the caring thinker's concern for humanity and justice and creates attitudes about the way things "ought" to be. In the realm of normative thinking, the caring thinker sees answers to problems and is frustrated when the problems go unsolved (e.g., bureaucratic red tape). In the face of lingering problems, the caring thinker continues to see the injustice and feel the pain and wants to intervene. He or she has passion, commitment, and a strong sense of ethics and values; society's values and expectations don't veer the caring thinker off course. This is likely why altruists are not deterred when individuals attempt to discourage their volunteerism. Their routine thinking is on a plane that is highly developed in terms of moral reasoning, empathy, justice, and decenteredness (rather than egoism).

A look at our twenty-two Good Samaritan organ donors causes us to speculate if they are indeed "gifted." It could be that a mind-set of caring thinking (in the setting of good health, economic stability, and psychosocial stability and support) is what sets Good Samaritan organ donors apart from those who are not donors. While we did not assess their IQ (intelligence quotient), our interviews are rich with information that correlates well with the four elements of caring thinking and, most specifically, the concepts of empathy, justice, and other-oriented vision. As children, 86 percent of our donors were troubled when they saw children being bullied or humiliated or if they saw violence in cartoons. As children, 62 percent of them sought out ways to correct injustice. Several expressed extreme frustration at the difficulty of giving an organ away. Their answer to the problem of the large transplant waiting list and organ shortage seemed "easy." They rationally deconstructed the problem and concluded that people have two kidneys but need only one, so one is given to someone (anyone) in need: problem solved. They were perplexed when some transplant centers refused their organ offers and were frustrated by how long the donation process took when their offer was accepted.

The notion of caring thinkers being other-oriented correlates well with the fact that for many Good Samaritan organ donors, there is no direct personal connection to transplantation (e.g., a family member or friend has experienced organ failure, dialysis, donation, or transplant). They are not operating from a personal emotional connection to the topic (not that this would be inappropriate) when they decided to donate. For others, a transplant stimulus event (e.g., reading an article about donation, watching a documentary about transplantation, or receiving a flyer about an unknown dying patient) stirs an empathetic response and moves them to donate. For 64 percent of our Good Samaritan donors, they had no personal connection to donation or transplantation. Their decision-making was clearly other-oriented because there was no emotional connection between the donation and a prior personal event in the donor's life. (For example, the donor was not responding out of a sense of emotional reparation or reciprocation.) Half of our donors (eleven of twenty-two) pursued donation on receiving some type of specific transplant stimulus such as those indicated above. We speculate that these stimulus events trigger empathy and action-taking responses to the injustice that is characteristic of caring thinking.

Throughout our book, we have covered a lot of ground in terms of analyzing what makes a Good Samaritan donor "tick": genetics, neurological pathways in the brain, parental modeling, spiritual prodding, values, and caring thinking. While Good Samaritan donors may appear saintly, such labeling is a very superficial commentary on who these people are and how their brains work. We think science and psychology should continue to explore these matters in an effort to explain the unknowns and calm some of the fears that society has about organ donation to strangers.

· 15 ·

Cynthia: A Valentine's Day Gift

Valentine's Day is typically filled with chocolate, fine wine, and filet mignon. On February 14, 2008 Cynthia's dinner table didn't bear any of those items, but it was still one of the most fabulous days of her life. In fact, Cynthia ate nothing on Valentine's Day because she was recovering from surgery. She had given a kidney to a stranger at New York-Presbyterian Hospital/Weill Cornell Medical Center.[1] This was the perfect Valentine's Day gift for her recipient, Anna Maria, who had been on dialysis for three years because of kidney failure caused by diabetes and high blood pressure.

It would be an understatement to say that Cynthia has a history of prosocial behavior.[2] She has been a routine blood donor and has been at the ready to donate bone marrow should she be identified as a match to someone in need. In addition, she is the eighth of eleven children, so sharing is second nature to her. As a child, she wanted to grow up to be a psychiatrist or a teacher (both helping professions) but eventually enlisted in the U.S. Marines. There, she worked her way up to the rank of sergeant and specialized in radio repair. Eventually, she became an accountant. Her love for the Marine Corps continued, literally, as she married a fellow Marine, Clint. He proved to be her role model for kidney donation because, in 1996, he donated one of his kidneys to his brother, who had end-stage renal failure due to diabetes.

Cynthia had wanted to be a living donor after seeing her husband go through the process with positive results. At the time, however, she had no friends or family members who were in need of a transplant, and the practice of Good Samaritan organ donation was in its infancy. "It's just something I've always wanted to do. . . . Living close to it in the family and seeing how well my brother-in-law did after the surgery—and he wasn't expected to live long on dialysis—was my motivation. I thought if I could do that for somebody else, and it wasn't going to physically affect me in the long run, why wouldn't I?"[3] But when she searched the Internet for hospitals that offered Good Samaritan organ donor programs, she found none. At the time, hospitals either were too afraid (minimally invasive techniques to remove kidneys did not exist yet) or did not have the procedures in place to handle Good Samaritan donations. So for eleven years, Cynthia's impending donation sat on the back burner until the medical profession was ready for her.

That day came along in 2007. Cynthia was watching television, and a documentary about organ donation appeared. She listened intently and learned that some transplant hospitals were now performing Good Samaritan organ donations using a laparoscopic (minimally invasive) procedure for kidney removal. Excited about the prospect of finally being able to donate, she contacted the National Kidney Registry, and they assembled their very first chain of donors and recipients.[4] In a chain donation, there are several people who need kidneys, and they all have willing living donors, but unfortunately the donors are not immunologically compatible with their friends/spouses/siblings/children. A Good Samaritan comes to the rescue and starts a living donation chain of events whereby all the donors get shuffled into compatible pairs (to patients they do not know). In this way, not only does the Good Samaritan donor help the patient who receives his or her organ, but the other patients get indirectly helped by the Good Samaritan because that's who starts the chain (facilitates its existence). In the United States, the National Kidney Registry helps arrange chain donations using their database of over 100,000 donor candidates and patients. Formed in 2008, the registry facilitated 200 transplants during its first twenty-two months.

Cynthia was ecstatic because as a chain donor, her donation would start a sequence of donations (like falling dominoes), so, in fact, she would be facilitating the transplants of several patients rather than just one. It didn't matter to her that she would need to fly from her home in California to the hospital in New York to accomplish the task. She was ready to pack her suitcase and head to the airport. And her husband gave his full support.

Many of Cynthia's medical tests were performed before she left home. The remaining tests were completed on arrival in New York. Like other donors, she was assessed by a social worker and a psychiatrist to ensure that her motives were altruistic and that there was no coercion or conflict of interest (e.g., seeking payment for her kidney). The donor team also wanted to ensure that she was fully informed and understood the procedure, its risks, and recovery issues. Cynthia was never fearful about donating: "If it's my time, it's my time."[5]

The surgeries were logistically complex, involving six surgical teams, six operating rooms, and forty clinical assistants. Cynthia did well and had no complications except for some nausea caused by the postoperative pain medication (not uncommon), which she discontinued when she realized she really didn't need it. Her pain was much less than she anticipated it would be, and her hospitalization was less than forty-eight hours. She has no regrets and would repeat her decision to donate if she had the opportunity. "I don't even miss the other kidney."[6] She is also proud of her scars.

Cynthia never had a desire to choose the recipient of her organ or even meet the individual. Her only goal was to help improve someone's life so that the person was no longer "tied down to machines."[7] Even so, with everyone's consent, all members of the chain (three donors and three recipients) met six days after surgery at the hospital. She states that when they initially gathered in the hospital waiting room, nobody knew who were the donors and who were the recipients. They had to be introduced to each other to learn their place in the chain. She describes her recipient as "the sweetest little thing" who is "very appreciative."[8] In spite of language differences, the recipient was clearly able to communicate her gratitude to Cynthia.

In the United States, thanks to the Department of Health and Human Services, February 14 is officially recognized as National Donor Day. It serves as an encouragement for individuals to remember patients in need and to consider participating in blood, marrow, stem cell, or organ donation. On this day, many employers offer blood drives where employees can gather at a central location and donate blood. Some employers promote organ donor registration with the assistance of their regional organ procurement organization, which provides education and enrollment materials. While Cynthia was moved to donate after witnessing her husband do the same, she indicates that she likely still would have been a living donor even if her husband had not. *Why?* "Giving is just important to me, and when I can, I will."[9]

· *16* ·

Ken: The "Life Preserver"

*K*en has a Mercedes, but it's not the kind you expect. It doesn't have four wheels, luxury leather, sleek styling, and an amazing sound system. Ken's Mercedes is also much more valuable than any vehicle. You can find his Mercedes on his abdomen: a large, three-pointed star-shaped scar. Just ask him to lift up his shirt. He's not shy. He's proud to show it off. He has also joined a regional club of liver donors who all bear this signature star. Ken, however, is a unique member of the club because he didn't donate liver tissue to a friend or relative—he gave it to a stranger.[1]

Ken, a highly talented artist,[2] is the son of an orthodontic technician father and factory worker mother. He is the middle of three children and evidences many prosocial behaviors. Thus, it shouldn't have been a shock to Virginia Commonwealth University's Medical College of Virginia Hospital in Richmond when he called them offering to give a lobe of his liver to a stranger. He'd already donated nearly twenty gallons of blood over the years (roughly the total amount of blood in fourteen adults). And, as a volunteer fireman, he had rescued people from roaring flames and delivered babies for their nervous parents. For Ken, living donation was just another form of altruistic behavior that made perfect sense to him. He was accustomed to putting his life on the line for others.

In reality, the hospital should have been waiting for Ken's call. The day before, a local television station ran a news story about a thirty-nine-year-old woman who needed a liver transplant. Her father was on the air, talking about her liver disease (hepatitis C contracted from a blood transfusion during gallbladder surgery). Ken, who doesn't normally watch much television, heard the story and knew he had the same blood type as the patient: B-positive. He also thought about his own daughter and the fact that if she ever had the same need, he hoped someone would assist their family. Within seconds, he made up his mind to donate and contacted the television station to initiate the process. A surprise to him, he was the only person to call. He assumed there would be lots of people coming forward with offers to donate.

The Virginia hospital had never performed a Good Samaritan liver donation before (no hospital had), and they were very nervous about doing so. They wondered if Ken was crazy or if he had motivations that weren't altruistic. The battery of psychosocial testing and consultations were extremely intense, to the point of irritating him. He feels he spent more time on the psychosocial screening than the medical screening. In the end, the donor team learned several things from Ken: he was not crazy, his motives were altruistic, and there *are* people in the world who "just like to do good things, and it's just that simple."[3] They also learned that it was simply the act of *helping* another person that mattered to Ken rather than the identity of the individual. "I couldn't let a stranger drown any easier than I could let somebody in my own family drown."[4] He's not a religious person or a philosopher; rather, he simply believes in treating others as he would want to be treated.

Deborah, the intended recipient, was overwhelmed by the generosity of her stranger donor. While she was excited about the prospect of a transplant, she was also worried that the donor might change his mind and back out at the last minute. Prior to their surgeries, both of them were at the hospital on the same day to have blood testing performed. In fact, they were in the waiting room at the same time when Ken's name was called to the nurse's desk, and she wondered if the mystery man might, in fact, be her donor. Deborah approached, tapped him on the shoulder, and asked him. Without hesitation, Ken admitted his donor status, and he received an incredible hug—"a hug like I'll never get again in my life."[5] He also reassured her that she could have any sort of worry she wanted to, but there was no need for her to worry about him changing his mind. "If I can do it, I'm going to do it, and it's that simple."[6]

From the start, Ken had the support of his wife and daughter. They even signed consent forms stating their agreement to his participation as a donor. As if on a strategic mission, Ken took his role as a donor very seriously. Two weeks prior to his surgery, he became very concerned about keeping himself in optimal health for the donation. He stayed home and kept himself away from anyone who was ill. He even refused to shake hands with people out of fear he might contract a cold or flu virus. He wanted to be in tip-top shape for Deborah. And he was. In April 1999, Ken gave his right liver lobe to Deborah. From then on, she referred to him as her "life preserver."[7] Even the living donation program director, Dr. Amadeo Marcos, was astounded: "I don't have words enough to say how incredible this gift is."[8]

Ken's only complication was a kidney stone, and it is unclear whether this was related to the surgical procedure. Looking back, Ken would repeat his donation "in a second."[9] As he told us, "People who have never done it . . . they don't know what they're missing!"[10] He encourages others to donate, and his experience, after it was publicized, resulted in three more living donations that he is aware of.[11]

Like most of the other Good Samaritan donors we interviewed, Ken was never fearful about the donation procedure. This might be partly due to the fact that Ken has lots of hospital experience. As a teenager, Ken was the victim of a tragic car accident and spent a year of his life in and out of the hospital. It was during this time, laid up, that he discovered his talents as a pencil artist, drawing beautiful illustrations. While his peers were running and playing football, he was using his creative energy and sketching. This is now his full-time occupation.

Unfortunately, Deborah died of kidney failure in 2008.[12] Ken's gift of a liver lobe enabled her to have eight years of life extension and the ability to witness the marriage of her daughter. As Deborah told him two days after the transplant, placing his hand where the graft was implanted, "He's got a sister now, and I've got another brother. We'll have this bond forever."[13] Ken will always have Deborah in his life.

• 17 •

Karen: Pay It Forward

$\mathcal{K}$aren's youthful appearance belies her fifty-five years. A married mother of three, her short, light brown hair brings out her dark eyes, which sparkle with fun and energy, making her seem like a woman twenty years younger. A successful insurance executive, she enjoys hiking and spending time with her family. But a few years earlier (during a period of temporary unemployment), she was asking herself, "What else can I do?"[1]

Karen knows a lot about risk, and she is a calculating thinker. For most of her life, she has worked in the field of insurance and risk management. And while she doesn't consider herself a risk taker, the fact that she has been a bone marrow donor *and* a kidney donor and that both recipients were strangers says a lot about Karen. *What gave her the comfort level to do these things? What motivated her?*

Karen witnessed prosocial behavior very early in her life. Her father served in the Army, and her mother was a nurse. As a child, Karen wanted a career as a social worker, but her path ultimately led her to the business world. Her activities with the United Church of Christ have positioned her well as an activist, as she does not believe in simply sitting back and praying or hoping that change will happen. Whether it is rallying stakeholders to come together and support energy efficiency (she has a passion for sustainability) or giving of herself (literally) to save a life, Karen makes change happen.

In 1995, a coworker asked Karen if she would participate in a bone marrow registration drive sponsored by her nephew's Boy Scout troop. Karen signed up and matched to two patients in need of a marrow transplant. One patient died before the transplant could happen, so Karen donated to the other patient. A year later, she met the recipient, and to this day she still receives birthday and Christmas cards from him. This positive experience, combined with her continuing good health, made her wonder what else she could do to save lives. Karen knew that living kidney and liver donation were possible, but she also knew that she was getting older, so her time line for clinical giving would be limited.

Watching television news reports, Karen had followed the donation story of another local Good Samaritan, Jack (also profiled in our book). His experience helped inform her about the kidney donation process and gave her comfort about the safety of the procedure. Doing her own research as well, she decided to pursue kidney donation, partly because the data show that kidney grafts last longer than liver grafts, and she wanted her donation to have significant impact for the recipient in terms of quality of life and life span of the transplant. It didn't matter that she wouldn't get to choose who received her gift and that possibly they would never meet. Karen has a mind for helping. In addition, her husband works for a hospital that has a world-renowned transplant facility, the Cleveland Clinic (the same hospital where Jack donated). The well-known integrity of the hospital gave her much confidence that she would be safe and well taken care of.

In 2007, with the support of her husband and children and after almost ten months of tests and clinical assessments (including a consultation with a clinical ethicist), Karen gave a kidney to a stranger at the top of the organ waiting list. Although the postoperative pain medication upset her stomach (this is common), she experienced no surgical complications and was discharged from the hospital in a few days. She still marvels at how small her scar is: "I don't understand how they could have gotten a kidney out of that!"[2] Several months later, she met the recipient of her kidney, a grateful man in his thirties who still occasionally calls her with progress reports. In 2010, he suffered a heart attack but recovered.

Looking back, she has no regrets about her decision to donate and would repeat her choice if she had the opportunity. She talks casually about her experience and does not brag to others. In fact, she doesn't mention it to others unless they bring up the topic. She promotes organ and marrow donation when asked but does not force the topic. For Karen, she believes that donation is her opportunity to "pay it forward" because she has had many blessings in her life.

V

LIFE EXPERIENCE
AND GIVING

· *18* ·

Altruism, Abundance, and Suffering

ALTRUISM BORN OF ABUNDANCE

*M*uch of the information we have presented up until now shows a form of altruism that is associated with personal bounty. What emerges from these individuals is something we term "altruism born of abundance." We boldly put forth this term to the community of transplant professionals as well as social science professionals so that they will have formal nomenclature to express what we have been deconstructing throughout this book. Our context is donation and transplant, but we feel that the terminology can carry to any domain, whether it involves goods, services, or information.

We define "altruism born of abundance" as altruistic motivations and acts that are realized by individuals who have reached a stage of contentment in their lives. "Abundance" does not necessarily mean material or financial wealth; rather, the state is personal contentment and satisfaction (and this may or may not involve wealth). Life has various segments, including education, career, mental and physical health, family, friends, finances, spirituality, and identity. Amid these segments, people will find a set of features that create their picture of life satisfaction. For some, the picture might include a doctoral degree, two children, and a wide circle of friends, whereas for others, it might be Zen-like living with no significant family ties. Whatever the recipe, at the core is a heart and mind that are fulfilled.

Looking at our Good Samaritan donor profiles, we find that 59 percent (thirteen of twenty-two) exhibited characteristics resembling altruism born of abundance. This is not to say that these individuals have a "perfect" life of serenity or that they have large bank accounts. In fact, most of the donors in this group had a moderate annual household income of $51,000 to $75,000 during the year in which they donated. What they all share is the common theme of

89

proclaiming that they are "blessed," "lucky," "fortunate," or desiring to give (or "give back") because they have plenty—their cup runneth over. For some, the mere fact of having two healthy kidneys (or a liver that can regenerate) equated to having more than they needed. These individuals thought it was no sacrifice at all to give a kidney away. For them, the second kidney was an extra that they had no need to keep. They didn't see it as something they required for daily living, and they looked for a way to put it in the hands of someone who could benefit from it. Operating from this philosophical platform, these individuals are keenly aware of their contentment and abundance and look outward to find a way to distribute their blessings (good health) to others.

Altruism born of abundance does not exclude other elements present and contributing to the desire to help others. For example, empathy is also commonly seen in these same individuals, and it is often what stimulated their desire to donate. Or they were emotionally touched by seeing or reading stories about living donation cases. On the opposite end of the emotional spectrum lies another sphere of altruism. It can precede, coexist with, or follow altruism born of abundance. This altruism arises from negative events such as trauma, hurt, and anguish.

ALTRUISM BORN OF SUFFERING

In 2003, psychologist Ervin Staub coined the term "altruism born of suffering."[1] This suffering can take many forms, such as that which is inflicted on the sole individual or a group of people, and the cause may be intentional (e.g., bullying, war, or rape) or unintentional (e.g., illness). In these situations, altruism occurs when an individual who experienced the suffering is able to move beyond it, transforming it so that the person turns *outward* in a helping manner toward others. On the surface, this is very simplistic, for there is much happening during that outward-turning process. Traumas can have deep and long-lasting negative effects, and these can inhibit a person from a positive attitude, "good" mood, or desire to help. Suffering people can be plagued with depression, anxiety, insomnia, loss of appetite, hopelessness, and nightmares. These can potentially cause more negative events (in addition to the original trauma), such as relationship troubles, job problems, and a decline in physical health. If one is sliding toward the dark side, how does the turnaround to an others-centered focus occur?

One approach is to look at time as a continuum rather than an isolated event. Viewing time as a continuum, there is a span of time that preceded the trauma and suffering. Exploring that span of time, there are several important things to look for that are potential moderators allowing a turnaround to an others-centered focus (the transformation of the trauma from a negative to a positive). These potential moderators include a personal prior history of pro-social behavior, adventurism, the sense of a responsibility for the well-being of others, parental modeling of prosocial behavior, the ability to empathize, an intolerance for injustice, recognizing that all humanity is one family, recognizing that all humanity has the same fate, an emotionally supportive environment, an optimistic personality, nurturing behavior, and strong coping skills. The presence of these moderators (before and after the trauma), as well as their strength or intensity, can help people transform their tragedies. Altruism can be an outgrowth of the suffering.

But lacking a prior history of altruism, how could altruism grow out of suffering? There might be something within the suffering event itself that is a trigger for the altruism—something that puts a positive spin on the negative situation. Maybe something was learned. Maybe a friend was made. Maybe enemies permanently left the scene. Maybe a foundational value system, such as one's religious beliefs, cast a special light on the suffering and gave it a purpose. Maybe the individual was able to see new meaning in his or her own life as a result of this suffering. Or maybe the altruistic act is a way of coping. The act of turning toward others means that individuals are no longer focused on themselves (and their suffering); instead, their focus is diverted to others.

Another interesting concept is the idea that observing the suffering of others can remind individuals of the suffering that they themselves experienced. Not only can this trigger empathy, followed by altruistic acts, but it can trigger a different path, namely, helping behavior toward others as a means to relieve one's own personal distress. An example of this is witnessing a dying child by way of either a newspaper article or a television news story. If the observer had a prior experience with a dying child (either his or her own illness as a child or the illness of his or her own child or sibling), this could stir up memories and physical and emotional distress. Hospitalizations are filled with many unpleasantries, such as needles, loud noises, pain, and medication side effects. Memories of illness-related suffering can be vivid, but so too can the memories about the help that was received along the way. These memories of the help and the helper may, in fact, contribute to a desire to step into that role. Because an individual has "been there," this can facilitate the stepping into the shoes of another. Looking toward the other person, the shoes look familiar, even painful, and there is a reminiscence of the shoes once worn. The experiential knowledge is a set of emotions, thoughts, and physical sensations. These can trigger empathy and move the individual to help. When this happens, the altruistic acts might relieve one's own suffering as well as another's. Further, there might be no overt intention of ministering to oneself; rather, it may come as an unintended consequence.

The most well-known studies of altruism born of suffering are those pertaining to the heroes of the Nazi era who sheltered or rescued Jews.[2] These helpers were often not Jews helping members of their own clan but simply those who could empathize or those who also felt ostracized in some way. Other studies on this topic have found altruism born of suffering emerging from the victims of terrorist attacks,[3] natural disaster,[4] sexual abuse,[5] illness,[6] and bereavement.[7] In our work, we identified three Good Samaritan organ donors whose experience resembles primarily altruism born of suffering: Josie, Garrett, and Arlene. Other donors, such as Matt and Jeff, also have elements of altruism born of suffering in their profiles, but parental modeling and destiny, respectively, appear as the driving themes.

As presented earlier, Josie's trauma was watching her partner of seventeen years slowly dying of renal failure in front of her on a daily basis. She watched him physically suffer the complications of kidney failure as well as the physical side effects of dialysis. Concurrently, she watched him emotionally suffer as his life changed shape over time. He went from an active sportsman to being unable to walk. He and Josie, together, faced up to an eight-year wait for a kidney. She made a move. She joined a donation chain, giving a kidney to a stranger so that her spouse could, in turn, receive a kidney, also from a stranger.

Garrett's full story will be presented in a subsequent chapter. His trauma was the death of his young wife. She was only thirty-four when she passed away from cancer. He remarried, and then his new wife was diagnosed with Hodgkin's disease. He was knocked down but not knocked out. He wasn't going to be an observer anymore; he was going to do something. And as many bereaved spouses do, he turned outward and performed prosocial behavior; namely, he gave a kidney to a stranger.

Arlene (whose donation was part of the inspiration for us writing this book) had several tragedies in her life, but they had a common theme: loss. Her father committed suicide when she was five years old. Her first husband became an alcoholic and committed suicide after Arlene left him. One of her brothers died in a biking accident, and another brother was murdered during a drug deal. During her second marriage, she found herself a single mother taking care of her husband's three children as well as the two they had together because her spouse walked out on her. Her altruism began with blood and platelet donation and continued to kidney donation to a stranger.

So, whether it's altruism born of suffering, abundance, genetics, personal moral duty, universal moral code, divine order, or another mechanism (or combination thereof), we desire that transplant professionals recognize the signs and not simply disregard those approaching them. Fear and ignorance should be replaced with knowledge and rational deliberation. We aim to pave a path for teams to walk on as they assess their donor candidates.

· 19 ·

Chad: Kidney-Shaped Cufflinks

$\mathcal{M}$ormons are known for their volunteerism. Between 1985 and 2007, members of the Church of Jesus Christ of Latter-Day Saints provided more than $1.01 billion in total humanitarian assistance to needy individuals in 165 countries.[1] Chad is one of those church members, but it is impossible to put a price on the value of his volunteerism. He gave one of his kidneys to a stranger and saved her life.

Chad pondered the idea of being a kidney donor for about three years before taking the steps to give his kidney to a needy patient.[2] He had heard about kidney donation on television and was aware that Utah Jazz basketball star Greg Ostertag had donated a kidney to his sister, then returned to the arena without a problem. He figured if Greg could return to professional basketball, then he could surely return to his public affairs job. After selecting from the two hospitals that perform living kidney donation in his home state, he approached University Hospital in Salt Lake City, Utah, and began his candidacy screening.

The psychiatrists were very interested in understanding Chad's personality and motivation for donating, so they subjected him to a battery of tests—more than 600 questions.[3] They wanted to be sure that he was mentally sound and was not selling his organ. In interviews, they probed him to find out what, specifically, was motivating his desire to donate. According to Chad, "The world seems like such a selfish place. Being a Good Samaritan Donor flies in the face of that. I've led a charmed life. I am healthy. I have a good job and family support."[4] He also has a history of prosocial behavior, such as blood donation and Boy Scout volunteering. Chad also states that he felt a spiritual confirmation to move forward with his decision to donate, but it did not spawn his decision—it confirmed it. Knowing that her husband is a "spiritual man," Chad's wife, Tracy, supported his decision to donate "without hesitation."[5]

Chad is the youngest of five children. Growing up, he had to deal with sharing one bathroom with four sisters. *That* challenge was a lot more difficult than sharing one of his kidneys with a stranger. The hospital's evaluation process was lengthy, but it was straightforward and ethically sound, matching his organ to the neediest patient. Chad had no desire to select a patient from among the thousands of compelling biographies posted on the Internet.[6] He liked the idea that his kidney would go to whomever the hospital felt needed it most. In fact, he had no desire to meet the recipient and was surprised to be presented with a consent form about the topic on the day of donation. "It wasn't even on my radar."[7]

Because Chad signed the consent form allowing contact between him and his recipient, he was able to meet her after surgery. While the transplant operation was without complication, the recipient got sick with a viral infection a few days after she left the hospital. This illness required her to return for care, and Chad went to the hospital to visit her and her family. In getting to know her, Chad found out that she had had some fears along the way (even though he had none). Specifically, she told him, "All I kept thinking was that you would probably change your mind any second and so even as I was shivering in my gown I refused to let myself get excited."[8] She was the only child of a single mother, so she had very few relatives and no matches for living donation. Chad was her lifesaver. He never had any doubts about his decision to participate, and he prepared himself well, including meeting other living donors beforehand and also watching a living donor surgery on the Internet.

Chad is clearly a thoughtful person. And he didn't forget about the care he received as a donor. He was very grateful to the donor team, especially his nurse, to whom he wrote a thank-you letter. With Chad's permission, we reprinted portions of his letter here:[9]

> Dear Transplant Nurse, . . . On October 5, 2007 I donated a kidney to someone I did not know. While I thought I had covered all the bases I had not thought much about those who would see me through those first painful and difficult days after surgery. While still very groggy from the anesthesia the first words I heard after surgery were from a transplant nurse who said, "You did a wonderful thing." My eyes were still closed so I didn't see her face and these simple words were whispered in my right ear as I was wheeled from the post-operative recovery room. It was a touching and intimate moment between a patient and care giver. The small things really count and I'll never forget it.

Chad had no complications after surgery other than a minor bladder infection that was easily treated with antibiotics. His life has returned to his usual work and exercise routines. Nine months after surgery, he even climbed Mount St. Helens. He also does regular hikes in Mount Zion National Park. If anyone complains during these excursions, he reminds them that *he* has only one kidney and he is doing just fine.[10] Even though his life has returned to normal, his daughter, Ali, considers her father a hero and has written a poem about him, the recipient, and a special thank-you present. With Ali's permission, we reprinted the full text of her poem here:[11]

> Kidney Shaped Cuff Links
> Once upon two years ago
> A man donated his kidney.
> To a young woman went the organ,
> She came from The Rocks of Sydney.
> Anonymous this was supposed to be,
> But the girl had something else in mind,
> For she wanted to meet this mystery man—
> The one who saved her from death's bind.
> So at Rainbow Gardens they finally did meet,
> His family and her close friend.
> Together they dined on delicious food
> Thankful it's no longer her end.
> When all were done eating and after chatting a while,
> The girl said she had something for him.
> Then out of her purse she pulled a small box,
> And out stretched her weak nimble limb.
> Slowly he opened the little blue package,
> "Tiffany's" read the gold brand name,
> And there in white velvet laid kidney-shaped cuff links,
> Shiny and silver they came.
> Two little cuff links, in a drawing of hands,
> Mean the world to the man's daughter—
> Who admires, through tear stained eyes,
> Her hero and best friend: her father.

Chad's donation touched several lives and it will continue to do so. For the recipient, not only did she get a new life, but she leapt forward to help others. A person with a graduate degree and a career in business and finance, her transplant experience placed her on a new career path: she quit her job and enrolled in medical school. Her plan is to become a transplant physician and use her personal encounter with illness, donation, and transplant to transform lives.

Chad's own words are the best summary of the story. "Living donation is something we truly have control over in ending the shortage of viable organs for those who are waiting and in many instances dying while they wait. . . . In my case, I was admitted on a Friday morning and left the hospital the following Monday morning. Since then my life has gone on without missing a beat—no physical limitations whatsoever. I'd do it again if I could."[12] And he was more than happy to talk with us about his donation experience. As he told us, "Too many people are needlessly suffering and dying waiting for a kidney. That won't change if people don't talk about it. Whether the motivation for donating is from a religious, humanitarian or some other perspective—the people waiting for a kidney don't care, they just want a shot at life and better health like all the rest of us."[13]

· 20 ·

Curt: Prunes and Motorcycles

$\mathcal{O}$ne look at Curt, and you realize that this is a person you want to get to know better. Spend five minutes with him, and you want to spend the whole day with him. The youngest of five children, Curt has a contagious smile, handsome looks, and an amazing wit. If he wasn't the vice president of human resources for one of the top ten ranked Fortune 500 companies in the United States, we think he could easily pursue stand-up comedy. When this forty-three-year-old from Dallas decided that he wanted to be a living liver donor, he was worried he might be rejected because he is gay. But, in fact, he proved to be healthy and was considered a perfect donor.

Curt is engaging and loves going out to discerning restaurants where he is a connoisseur of wine and martinis. In fact, his love of martinis had him a little concerned that his liver might not be suited for donation (and that he might not be able to partake afterward), but neither materialized. While Curt likes some of the finer things in life, he considers himself somewhat of a "nerd."[1] His favorite magazines are *Popular Mechanics*, *Popular Science*, and *Car and Driver*. He also loves to watch science-fiction movies, and his favorite mode of transportation is a Harley-Davidson. He says of himself, "I have a love of all things science and gadget-related. My close friends just shake their heads."[2]

Working in upper management, Curt does a lot of business travel. Curt does so much travel that he cannot remember where he was going or where he was coming from when he was airborne 30,000 feet in 1999, reading a newspaper story about a mother who donated a portion of her liver to her toddler. Because he loves science, the story fascinated him. He was intrigued to learn that the liver could be cut into pieces and regenerate. He was "captivated."[3] The scientist portion of Curt's brain spoke and said, "Well if this can be done, why is everybody dying? Why can't people just give part of their

97

liver to [other] people?" Curt's logic was that more than 15,000 people a year were dying of liver disease, yet the technology to stop those tragedies was available: living donation.

Curt could not get the concept out of his mind. He went to the Internet and searched for a transplant hospital with which he could arrange a liver lobe donation. He found three places: one in Japan and two in the United States (Pittsburgh and Los Angeles). Japan was too far away—so he excluded that hospital. Same for Pittsburgh. Los Angeles seemed the best fit for him because he actually knew the hospital (University of Southern California), as they were a business client. In addition, he was familiar with the area because he had made numerous trips to the city in the past. While Curt may have selected the hospital, would *they* select him? The rest of the donation process was not as easy.

Initially, the hospital was suspicious. This was because the concept of Good Samaritan liver donation hadn't come up before at their facility. Other donors were either friends or relatives of the recipients. Curt's inquiry came with no recipient in tow. He wanted to give to a stranger, possibly a child, but really anyone in need. The hospital's ethics department was in a quandary. As Curt describes the situation, "They were freaked out. They didn't know what to do with the whole thing. . . . All I wanted to do was to help somebody."[4] At the time, unbeknownst to Curt, the hospital was perplexed at how to respond to his request, and the staff volleyed their concerns back and forth among themselves. Back then, there had been only one Good Samaritan liver donor in the world, but Curt didn't know that and didn't understand the cautionary tone of the situation. According to Curt, the hospital increased their comfort level by having him assessed by several psychiatrists. Passing those evaluations and the medical screenings (including multiple HIV tests to verify his negative status), the hospital allowed the donation to proceed.

While Curt may have put to rest the concerns held by the hospital, his mother and best friend were not singing his praises. Admitting that living donation is an admirable act, both were frightened that he might become injured (or die) as a result and preferred that he change his mind and not participate. Yet, while he loves and respects both of these people, Curt would not back down. "I was bound and determined I was gonna do this."[5]

Curt recovered in the hospital for a week and then continued his recovery at a local hotel for another two weeks before returning home. His recovery was not uneventful. In addition to the barrage of media, he battled chronic nausea, which relented only after several months (and a steady diet of prune juice). It's no surprise that the lengthy battle with nausea caused him to experience depression, as his quality of life during that time was miserable. He also spent about $9,000 of his own money to accomplish the donation because at the time there were no financial grants for living donors (for travel, lodging, meals, and so on) Even now, ten years later, there are negative comments on his credit report that pertain to hospital billing charges arising from the confusion of being a pioneer living donor. He calls his credit "a mess" but has no regrets about being a donor.[6]

Curt had a rocky recovery, and so did his recipient, Ray. Unfortunately, Ray lived for only a few months following transplantation. The liver transplant had been a success, but Ray caught a cold while immunosuppressed, and it advanced to pneumonia. This was devastating for Curt, who had developed a close relationship with both him and his family. Curt was given the honor of writing and speaking the eulogy at the funeral and retains the pall, a family gift, in memory.

Curt summed up Good Samaritan donation very succinctly: "If you want to be a Good Samaritan, I really believe you ought to decide to save a life, not a particular image of what you think a worthy life is . . . there was no reason why one life would be more important to me than the other."[7] Indeed, Curt and his recipient couldn't be more opposite. Curt is a George Bush Republican, white, and Methodist, while Ray was a Democrat, Hispanic, and Catholic. If people were image grading, they might have questioned if Curt's recipient should have gotten a liver at all because he was a former alcoholic who had acquired hepatitis C from homemade tattoos. None of this was ever on Curt's radar, and he likes that it happened that way (not knowing the patient beforehand and not meeting until afterward). Thanks to Curt, his recipient got another four months of life with his family. "You can't even believe how much fun he was having."[8]

Curt is brutally honest about the negative aspects of his donation and gives people fair warning that the surgery is "tough," but he has no regrets about his donation and would repeat his decision to participate if he had the chance. If people are expecting media praise, he advises them that the days of living donation hoopla are over. It shouldn't be the goal of donation, and people shouldn't sit awaiting the limelight grandeur. He's proud and excited to have been a donor, but he is honest with people when explaining his experience. It wasn't easy, and when his recipient died, he experienced a yearlong bout of depression.

Today, Curt enjoys his leisure time with the love of his life, Ellie, an Isabella dachshund. His best friend is relieved that Curt is safe and sound after donation, and the two of them ride motorcycles together (a gift from Curt) when time permits. Curt is a generous soul. Giving is part of his nature. When asked what he would want if he could have anything in the world, he replied, "The sense that my family and friends have what they need."[9] He would like to see his family and friends financially secure with no home mortgage.

He would also like to see Good Samaritan donation continue to happen but without the heavy veil of suspicion that he encountered. According to Curt, his recipient is the "most important person in this whole story,"[10] but people always seem to focus on Curt's heroics. As Curt told us, "It may not seem or be easy to explain, but in someone's head, their heart, they just want to do this . . . like for me it made absolute perfect sense . . . I literally, honestly . . . you can look me in the eye . . . why wouldn't I do this?"

Garrett: Helping the Vulnerable

$\mathcal{A}$s a prosecuting attorney with more than thirty years of legal experience, Garrett is a tough man to contend with. He helped put a man in prison who had used a shock collar as a form of punishment on his three children.[1] In another case, he sent a man to jail for predatory sexual behavior with a minor on the Internet.[2] Issues such as drug possession and burglary are also right up his alley. But Garrett has another side to him—warm, compassionate, and giving. In 2005 at age fifty-eight, he gave a kidney to a stranger, an African American teenage boy in a single-parent home with a life complicated by renal failure, autism, and other medical issues.[3]

Garrett is very familiar with the concept of suffering.[4] He served four years in the U.S. Army, two of which were spent in Vietnam during the war. Part of his military duties included escorting the bodies of deceased soldiers home to their families. He watched his father die of Alzheimer's disease, and his thirty-four-year-old wife die of cancer. After he remarried, his new wife was diagnosed with Hodgkin's disease. According to Garrett, he could no longer just sit back and be an "observer."[5] He wanted to do something to alleviate human suffering, so he searched the Internet for various opportunities. He'd already been involved in blood donation and other prosocial activities. After exploring several options, he determined that kidney donation was the "best thing that I could do,"[6] and he felt it was relatively safe. He spent a lot of time researching the donation procedure and then called several transplant hospitals in his region to ask about their programs. Eventually, he selected the Cleveland Clinic to begin his candidacy assessment.

No different from the other donors we interviewed, Garrett was intensely assessed by the hospital about his donation motives. *Why was a man with a doctorate, successful career, and happy family wanting to have a surgery he didn't need?* For Garrett, donation was all about the help he could provide. With a surgery that he prospectively viewed as not life altering for himself, he could provide someone else a great benefit in terms of improved quality of life. He had no desire to choose the recipient of his kidney or even meet the person. His wife and three children supported his decision but expressed concern for his safety, as most family members do, but they never tried to talk him out of it or steer him to another type of volunteerism. And like most Good Samaritan donors, he had no fears about the surgery (except worrying about the ever-present risk that it could get canceled if there was a complication with the intended recipient).

On a Thursday in April, Isaiah got a new kidney. The gift from Garrett put an end to his six years of dialysis. As a teenage boy, it certainly was a relief to no longer spend hours attached to a machine, watching his blood cycle through tubes. Isaiah's mother was a big part of the transplant process, for she was instrumental in helping him prepare. Autistic children have cognitive difficulties as well as impaired social development and communication skills; thus, a solid organ transplant can be emotionally and psychologically stressful for these patients and their caregivers. In fact, medical literature reports only one case of a transplant (a bone marrow transplant) in an autistic individual, and it required several weeks of educational and psychological preparation by the medical team.[7]

Two days after donation, Garrett left the hospital without complications and the following month had rode 900 miles on his bicycle. He's not kidding when he says, "I've always been blessed with good health."[8] Unfortunately, Isaiah didn't fare as well as his donor, contracting a virus six months after transplant that wiped out his new graft by the summer of 2006. He has returned to dialysis and awaits another transplant in the future. While Garrett is disappointed at the outcome, he has no regrets about donating. "Without question"[9] he would repeat his decision, and the boy's mother considers Garrett her "hero."[10]

Garret doesn't actively broadcast the events of donation, but he is happy to talk about the subject when others bring up the topic. In addition, he is at the ready as a mentor to living donor candidates to help them understand the screening process and answer questions they have along their assessment journey. Even though the success of his donation was time limited, Garrett is satisfied by the fact that each day he wakes up knowing that he made a positive impact on someone's life for a period of time. "Everybody is my brother and sister. . . . We have to get along and take care of each other when we can."[11]

VI

BECOMING AN
ORGAN DONOR

· 22 ·

Candidacy Evaluation

$\mathcal{T}$he process of becoming a Good Samaritan organ donor often surprises people. Many think that it is as simple as calling or emailing a transplant hospital and informing them of the desire to donate and a surgery date will be scheduled within days. One of our donors thought she could have the whole thing done and her recuperation completed (surreptitiously) while her husband was gone on a hunting trip.[1] For many good reasons, the evaluation process has several steps and takes time, often several weeks or months to accomplish. The donor team is a multidisciplinary group of individuals that works with the transplant team but is separate from them. The reason for this is to help ensure objectivity and limit opportunities for conflict of interest. Without interference from the transplant team, the donor team makes decisions about who is or is not acceptable to donate an organ. The two teams can network together to discuss matters of donor–recipient compatibility (e.g., immunology and anatomy), but they maintain their separate identity and autonomy.

TELEPHONE SCREENING

Once an individual (adult age eighteen or older) informs a transplant hospital of the desire to be a donor, the evaluation process begins with a telephone screening. During this phone call, a nurse (known as a transplant coordinator) asks the individual a series of questions pertaining to medical and psychosocial issues that are absolute exclusions to donating. For example, information about a person's height and weight lead to a calculation of body mass index (BMI). If the BMI is too high (>35 kg/m²) or too low (<18 kg/m²), the individual is automatically excluded as a donor because of elevated surgical risk. Females who are pregnant are also excluded. A personal history of struvite kidney stones (or other relevant kidney problems), high blood pressure (>140/90), diabetes, and certain heart problems also rule out donor candidates. Other issues, such as financial problems and current serious mental illness, exclude candidates as well because the stress of donation can exacerbate matters. In addition, these issues can potentially be a signal that the person is seeking donation for inappropriate reasons. Certain types of active mental illness can also pose problems during postdonation surgical recovery (e.g., compliance with medical advice).

The use of illicit drugs excludes candidates, as does cancers occurring within five years of the planned donation. All forms of cancer affecting the organ to be donated are contraindicated, even if the cancer was treated and has been in remission for more than five years. Alcohol addiction and abuse are also contraindicated. Those who smoke tobacco must agree to stop and must have satisfactory lung function. Similarly, if a candidate has hepatitis or HIV, this also excludes organ donation. Some U.S. transplant hospitals also require that the donor candidate have a personal health insurance policy even though the evaluation and surgery is paid for by the recipient's insurance. This is because if there is a medical complication, the recipient's insurance will pay for the expenses for only a limited time. If the complication is of a long duration or appears late after surgery (months or years), the donor will generally have to use personal means to pay the associated treatment costs. Some transplant hospitals also ask questions pertaining to citizenship to ascertain if there are any immigration problems that put the individual at risk of deportation to his or her home country (where the donor might not have access to suitable medical care). Candidates who are on parole are usually excluded from participating because of the risk of returning to prison (where health care quality and access can be poor).

Some transplant hospitals have upper age limits for living donation (e.g., age sixty), while others do not. In the United States, about 1.5 percent of living kidney donors are age sixty-five or older. We are aware of several cases of successful kidney donation from donors over age seventy.[2] These donors were otherwise very healthy and thus good candidates with low surgical risk. If the individual passes the telephone screening, plans are made for in-person medical and psychosocial screenings. The entire process may be slightly different at one transplant hospital compared to another, as there are few rigid rules about living donation and many relative (flexible) criteria. This said, transplant centers define their own policies and procedures for screening donor candidates.

PSYCHOSOCIAL SCREENINGS

Some transplant hospitals require that all living donor candidates be evaluated by a psychologist, while others use a psychiatrist for the process. This is in *addition* to the evaluation conducted by a social worker. Some use a combination of all three personnel to evaluate candidates, especially in situations of Good Samaritan donation or situations where there is suspicion of active mental illness. During the social worker's evaluation, the donor candidate is probed about matters such as financial stability, employment and insurance status, domestic relationships (life with spouse/partner), motivation for donation, conflict of interest, organ selling, coercion, and emotional health. The social worker will also evaluate the suitability of the candidate's social support system. This involves interviewing the designated support person (usually the candidate's spouse or life partner) to ascertain if the individual is content with the donation and if he or she is prepared to undertake the role as caregiver and provider for a limited time. Psychologists and psychiatrists take a deeper look at the emotions and behaviors of the individual. This can be done via personal interview, but sometimes these clinicians also administer oral and/or written psychological tests to explore the candidate's personality. If there is a question about the candidate's cognitive ability, neuropsychological testing can be done to determine if there is a deficit, what it involves (e.g., memory, concentration, problem solving, or language expression), and potential causes (e.g., stress, medication, injury, or disease).

Some transplant hospitals require that living donor candidates be assessed by a transplant ethicist. This is usually reserved for complex cases (e.g., where there is concern about ambivalence, organ selling, or conflict of interest) or cases involving Good Samaritan organ donation (because there is no emotional relationship between the donor and the recipient). This extra layer of assessment is a form of due diligence by transplant hospitals, evidencing that they look after the safety and welfare of donors as well as the integrity of their program and the practice of living donation in general. As a transplant ethicist, I (Dr. Bramstedt) have assessed dozens of living kidney and liver donor candidates. On occasion, I encounter ethical red flags, such as people who do not have altruistic motivations and those who have lied during their assessments. One of my most memorable cases was a man who was seeking to donate a kidney to a stranger he met through an Internet chat room. My assessment determined that he had recently been released from U.S. federal prison for wire fraud.[3] In another case, I evaluated a man who sought to be a living kidney donor to a stranger he met via an online social networking site intended to match donors and recipients. He had been seeking free medical care in our hospital emergency room under the pretense of his intent to be a living donor. He also was requesting money from the hospital, alleging that he had been mugged. My assessment revealed that this donor candidate had a lengthy criminal history and had been released from parole in his home state only a few weeks prior. In another state, he was reported as "absconded." His multiple crimes included convictions for check fraud, auto burglary, larceny, and forgery.[4]

MEDICAL SCREENINGS

There are numerous medical screenings that take place during the evaluation of living donors. This is to protect the safety of the living donor and to also ensure that the organ donated is healthy and safe for the recipient. If a living donor has disease (such as cancer or active infections), it is possible to transmit these to the recipient. Risk of transmission is extremely high, as recipients have weakened immune systems because of the antirejection medications they take (immunosuppressants).

Transplant hospitals start the medical screening process with very simple, low-risk tests. If the candidate passes these, the process advances to higher-risk tests. For example, the first tests that are done are blood and urine tests. A sample of blood is tested for a variety of parameters, including cell content (a complete blood count), blood type (ABO screening), ability to clot, pregnancy test for women, prostate-specific antigen test for men older than forty (to screen for prostate cancer), enzymes and other molecules that denote liver function, fat content, syphilis, HIV and hepatitis, and other chemistries. A sample of blood will also undergo HLA (human leukocyte antigen) testing in order to identify immunologic compatibility with potential recipients. Donors do not have to match their recipients in terms of race or gender, but their tissues must be compatible. A small sample of urine is examined for various features including infection as well as sugar and protein content. If stones are seen, these will be sent for chemical analysis. If the candidate is intending to donate a kidney, a collection of all the individual's urine produced in a twenty-four-hour period is saved and given to the laboratory for analysis. The lab will measure the urine volume and determine how well the kidneys work in terms of processing protein and creatinine.

Other simple tests that are performed include tuberculosis screening (skin test), chest X-ray, and an electrocardiogram. The latter measures the electrical activity of the heart and can detect an acute heart attack as well as heart rhythm disturbances and problems, such as low potassium and elevated calcium. Women older than forty will also need to have a mammogram and PAP smear testing performed (or recent results given to the transplant hospital for review).

If all these test results are normal, the donor candidate can proceed to a radiologic study of the abdomen and pelvis (potential kidney donors) or abdominal CAT scan and computed tomography cholangiogram (potential liver donors). During the cholangiogram, a dye is injected into the bloodstream so that the doctor can see the gallbladder and other areas where bile flows. The photographs taken allow the doctors to inspect for blockages, masses, and anatomical features. During the computed tomography of the abdomen and pelvis, doctors inspect the area blood vessels. These tests are painless but require the donor candidate to receive contrast dye. Side effects are rare, but there is the remote risk of having a serious allergic reaction to the dye (unconsciousness, shock, and/or death). Radiologic technicians are readily prepared for this type of emergency.

Some donor candidates might need additional testing, depending on their medical history. Men over age fifty will need to have a colonoscopy (or provide recent results to the transplant hospital for review). Other potential tests include cardiac stress testing (running on a treadmill), echocardiogram (external photography of the heart using sound waves), and ambulatory blood pressure monitoring (continual blood pressure monitoring for twenty-four hours to assess variability in pressures throughout the day). For those planning lung, pancreas, or intestinal donation, additional tests will be performed.[5]

In addition to the tests, a donor candidate is examined by a doctor (e.g., a nephrologist if donating a kidney, a hepatologist if donating a liver lobe, or a pulmonologist if donating a lung lobe) and a surgeon. Both clinicians review the medical data and physically examine the candidate. During this time, the candidate is prodded from head to toe to ensure that he or she is a good candidate. Questions are asked of the candidate to verify that there are no current or prior conditions that significantly increase the risk of general anesthesia, surgery, and postoperative recovery. (The candidate will also be further interviewed by an anesthesiologist after a surgery date has been scheduled.) The candidate's family history is queried in detail to ensure that there are no patterns of disease affecting the organ intending to be donated. Review of the imaging studies (pictures) and information about any prior surgeries helps the surgeon plan the donation (or decide against it). Both clinicians also assess the attitude, stress level, and motivation of the candidate (as the other team members did). They inform the candidate of the details of the donation procedure and its risks and benefits and evaluate if the candidate understands the information presented. If there is any uncertainty about the individual's capability to give informed consent, this is a red flag of concern, and neuropsychiatric testing may be needed. The candidate must have the capacity to give voluntary informed consent or the donation cannot occur.

Women who seek to be living donors are advised to stop the use of hormone-based contraceptives, as these can increase the risk of perioperative stroke. They are also counseled about postdonation pregnancy. In general, the data on this topic are minimal, but from what is known, there are concerns in two areas. In studies that were conducted in Norway[6] and the United States,[7] it was discovered that women who had been living donors and then subsequently became pregnant experienced slightly higher rates of preeclampsia (high blood pressure and increased excretion of protein into urine) and gestational high blood pressure than those who had not been donors. The U.S. study also identified higher rates of gestational diabetes.[8] While the Norwegian study identified no differences in stillbirths, neonatal mortality, preterm delivery, and low birth weight between the groups of births after kidney donation, before kidney donation, and the control group (a random sample of mothers),[9] the U.S. study observed a higher risk for fetal loss in women who were donors, but these women were also noted to be older.[10] It has been speculated that the increased risk for complications may be due to the burden of pregnancy imposed on a single kidney, and this might be analogous to the burden of multifetal pregnancy on women with two kidneys.[11] More research is needed on this topic, as the data currently available are limited. Women who are considering pregnancy after donation should talk to the nephrologist as well as their gynecologist to educate themselves as much as possible regarding potential risks. They might want to speak with women who have experienced pregnancy and childbirth after kidney donation. The donor team social worker can make these networking arrangements.

MISATTRIBUTED PATERNITY

Living donor candidates should be aware of the risk that blood testing performed during the screening process could *potentially* reveal misattributed paternity. These situations can arise when a donor candidate is screened to donate to a presumed relative but ABO and HLA blood tests reveal information that gives *indications* that the intended recipient might not be a genetic relative (e.g., a child and parent are not biologically related). It has been estimated that among living kidney donations between a father and presumed biological child, the prevalence of misattributed paternity is between 1 and 3 percent in the United States and Canada.[12]

It's important to note that transplant physicians, while they are very knowledgeable about medicine, are not experts on genetics. The testing that they do when they screen donor candidates is for the purpose of determining eligibility for donation. They have no role, clinically or psychosocially, to verify or refute parentage. The ABO and HLA testing that is done in the setting of a donation evaluation gives only limited information about parental assignment. In order to fully understand one's parentage, a full panel of genetic tests, interpreted by a board-certified genetic counselor, is required. The donor team can arrange referrals for these tests and consultations if the donor candidate provides consent.

LIVING DONOR ADVOCATE

In the United States, regulations require all transplant centers to have either an independent living donor advocate or an independent living donor advocate team.[13] The purpose of this role is to ensure that the donor/donor candidate always has someone to turn to for objective and unbiased information and counseling about donation. I (Dr. Bramstedt) have worked in such a role for several years on behalf of many kidney and liver donors. The advocate can originate from virtually any educational background, but most commonly these individuals have advanced degrees in subjects such as medicine, law, ethics, psychology, theology, and social work. They have additional training in transplant and donation in order to have the knowledge needed to converse appropriately in the matters at hand. The advocate can have a powerful voice at a transplant hospital. Advocates assess all living donor candidates and provide written reports to the donor team stating whether the candidates are suitable to participate as donors. The assessment explores the motivation for donation, level of willingness to donate, knowledge about donation, possible sources of coercion to donate, and so on. In general, if an advocate vetoes a candidate, the donor team accepts this opinion and stops the process (unless there are steps the candidate can take to rectify the shortcomings). The advocate will also inform the team if the candidate decides to decline to participate. At some transplant hospitals, the advocate also checks on the donor after surgery to ensure their wellness and to ascertain if any needs exist.

DONOR SELECTION COMMITTEE

After all the testing has been completed and all the clinicians have written their evaluation reports, the donor selection committee meets to review the information as a group and render a decision as to whether the candidate can participate as a living donor. The committee is a multidisciplinary group of professionals, consisting of transplant doctors and surgeons, nurses (transplant coordinators), social workers, the living donor advocate, a psychologist, a psychiatrist, and a financial coordinator. If the team has an ethicist, this individual also participates in case reviews and discussions.

A candidate might be clearly acceptable (medically and psychosocially healthy with appropriate motivation and no coercion) or unacceptable (medically unsafe, psychosocially unstable, inappropriate motivations, and/or coerced). Sometimes, a candidate can become acceptable if certain conditions are met (e.g., after losing ten pounds). Whatever the decision, it is made by committee consensus and then transmitted to the individual in writing. A copy of the letter is also placed in the individual's medical chart. If the individual was found unacceptable, an appeal can be made to the committee for reconsideration. The appeal should be made in writing and should indicate the reasons why re-review is requested. If the committee affirms its decision and the individual still has a strong desire to be a donor, contact can be made with another transplant hospital in an attempt to initiate another candidacy evaluation. In these situations, it is customary for the individual to be asked permission for sharing of the medical chart, as this prevents the candidate from having to repeat most tests and procedures already recently completed. The transplant hospital will also be able to review information pertaining to the individual's prior disqualification. While individuals may be disappointed at disqualification, the decision is for their safety and welfare. These matters are the primary concerns of the donor team (no matter the good intentions of organ donation).

Because disqualified individuals are considered patients with a medical record, their medical information is confidential and not disclosed to intended recipients. The only notification that the organ failure patient receives is the fact of the candidate's disqualification. They are not given any specific information with regard to the details (medical, psychosocial, or ethical matters).

ALMOST TO THE FINISH LINE

Once the candidate is approved for donation, the individual must sign a consent form. This form provides written details about the procedure as well as its risks and benefits. It also reminds the individual that the procedure is completely voluntary and warns against organ vending (selling the organ). After the form is signed, the individual receives a copy, and a "cooling-off" period begins. Most (but not all) transplant hospitals require a cooling-off period for their living donations. During this time, usually two to four weeks, individuals are asked to reflect on the decision to donate and given the opportunity to revoke their prior consent (change one's mind). Sometimes during this period, individuals gather additional information (or questions) about donation. Sometimes they meet with others who have been living donors in order to get firsthand experiential information. During this cooling-off period, there might also be a "homework" requirement for the individual, such as smoking abstinence. Individuals will be toxicology tested (urine sample) at random intervals before donation to ensure compliance with smoking cessation.

After the cooling-off period elapses, the individual is asked to sign the consent form a second time (to reaffirm their decision to donate). At any point in time, even on the day of surgery, while being wheeled into the operating room, individuals can revoke their consent, and the donation will be canceled. No specific reason needs to be given to the nurse or doctor. The ethical principle of autonomy allows individuals their free choice. The intended recipient will *never* be told the reason why the surgery was canceled, as these matters remain part of the confidential medical record of the other party. Usually, the patient is told that the donor team feels that the individual is no longer a suitable candidate in terms of safety or welfare. It is unethical to give a specific fake medical excuse ("He just had a minor stroke"), as this can cause alarm for the intended recipient, and if the fake medical excuse were to be placed in the medical chart, it could potentially have negative ramifications in terms of insurance risk profiling.

· 23 ·

The Donor's Family Circle

$\mathscr{P}$erhaps poet Sir John Donne said it best: "No man is an island."[1] People don't exist by themselves; rather, they are interconnected. They are spouses, partners, parents, aunts/uncles, siblings, employees, employers, mentors, coaches, friends, customers, clients, and patients. Nowhere is this interconnectedness more evident than in the specialty of transplant medicine. It is unlike any other clinical specialty in that it takes an alliance of people to make success happen—success for the living donor and success for the organ recipient. A good analogy is baseball. Everyone on the team needs to show up for practice promptly, wearing their uniforms, tools on hand (bat, ball, glove, and protective gear), agreeing to play by the rules, with an attitude that says, "Let's win."

In transplant and donation, the team members are the doctors, surgeons, nurses, financial coordinators, dieticians, social workers, psychologists, psychiatrists, ethicists, donor, recipient, and the families of the donor and recipient. Clearly, the family members of the organ recipient are critical because they help care for the patient after surgery and provide encouragement during rocky times (e.g., medication side effects, surgical complications, and organ rejection). Overall, family is often the reason that patients seek transplant—they want to resume the quality of life that they once had so that they can interact with their family and enjoy family life. *What, then, is so important about family in the setting of living organ donation? Isn't this a donor's decision to make? An autonomous choice?*

SPOUSES AND LIFE PARTNERS

Zell Kravinsky is likely the most famous case of a Good Samaritan donor who lacked family support.[2] In fact, Zell had asked a friend to create an alibi for him that would allow him to sneak away from his house for a few days so that he could donate a kidney to a stranger at Albert Einstein Medical Center in Philadelphia—all this because his wife (a psychiatrist) was not in favor of his extreme charitable giving. In fact, organ donation was just one in a series of major philanthropic events for Zell, including giving away almost his entire $45 million real estate fortune to charity. Lacking the cooperation of his friend, Zell decided to slip out of his house one summer morning in 2003 while his wife and children were still asleep and proceed with organ donation. His wife found out when she read a media report in a local newspaper. Zell gave away things (money and kidney) because he thought other people needed them. As he told *The New Yorker*, "With each thing I've given away, I've been more certain of the need to give more away. And at the end of it maybe I will be good."[3] (Comments like these should be red flags for psychosocial teams who evaluate living donor candidates, as they potentially signal an individual's misguided search for personal value and acceptance.) His wife expressed her view that their *own* family should come first and that he was taking too many risks, but Zell put the outside world as his priority. She also knew Zell's medical history and felt that his gastrointestinal problems made him a poor donor candidate. These matters caused considerable marital and family strife. The hospital was aware of Zell's lack of support but allowed his donation to proceed on the basis of personal autonomy—he was making a voluntary, informed choice, and he had the cognitive capacity to make his own decisions.

Zell's situation is not an isolated case of lack of familial support. A hospital in Minnesota reported a series of Good Samaritan kidney donors.[4] Two donors who were under age twenty-one had not told their parents of their donation until afterward because initially, when they spoke to their parents about the concept, they received negative reactions. (So as not to disrupt their donation plans, both donors had lied to the hospital, stating that their parents were approving of their wish to donate.) After donation, these two individuals were distressed about the prospect of informing the family of what they had done, not to mention the fact that they were without their parents as support persons at the time of surgery. The team also became aware, after donation, that spouses of three donors also voiced negative reactions to the concept at some point during the process. Similar to the cases of the young donors, two of these donors had lied to the hospital and indicated that their spouses concurred with their desire to donate. This hospital no longer allows Good Samaritan donation from individuals under age twenty-one even though the legal age for medical decision making is eighteen. While they strongly encourage family to attend the evaluation process along with the donor, they do not require it and do not require spouse/partner consent for the donation to proceed.

A donor needs a support system of some type. This is because donation requires the help of others, most significantly while the donor recovers from surgery. In the immediate postoperative period, the donor is still in the hospital setting, so he or she is assisted by nurses and others when needing to walk or reach for things. When discharged home, donors will need help for a least the near term. For example, they won't be able lift grocery bags (and they won't be driving to the grocery store to shop right away) and infants. Trips to the bank and pharmacy may be needed, and the donor might not feel up to it. In addition, others in the family may take on new roles for a while. If the donor was in charge of family chores like mowing the lawn and washing the car, someone else is going to have to do these activities for a period of time. If the donor drove the school carpool, someone else will need to assume that duty as well. Cooking, laundry, and housecleaning will all need to be reassigned temporarily.

If the donor was a breadwinner (or the sole provider of financial support), unpaid time away from employment can potentially put economic pressure on other members of the family to provide financial support or make financial concessions. The donor's spouse or life partner usually takes on extra caretaking duties in both that role and others, such as parenting. Because the donor's physical functioning is impaired during the recovery process, the role(s) once performed is temporarily changed, and other people fill in the gaps.

Another reason why living donation does not occur in a vacuum is that the decision can have far-reaching effects to members of the donor's family. Specifically, there are four matters that the donor and donor's family should consider together: 1) life insurance, 2) health insurance, 3) donor death or morbidity (complications), and 4) surrogate decision making. Unfortunately, with any surgery there is no crystal ball and no way to predict the outcome, so the best plan is to be prepared for any eventuality.

With regard to insurance, many individuals who seek to be living donors in the United States lack their own personal health insurance. Some transplant centers refuse to consider uninsured candidates; however, others will allow them to participate, with strong warnings that late-appearing side effects or those of long duration might not be covered by the organ recipient's medical policy. It is customary for the recipient's insurance to pay for the donor's medical complications, but they generally do so for only a limited time. In addition, the time period varies among insurance companies and can be as short as three months postoperation. We strongly advise all those who are considering participating as living donors to obtain their own health insurance. Even if donation does not happen, insurance is at the ready—an important consideration in the United States, where health care costs are among the highest in the world. Additionally, waiting to obtain health insurance until after donation can sometimes result in higher premiums.[5]

Donors and their families should also consider the matter of life insurance. While it is rare, there is always the risk of a donor dying as a result of living donation (either during or after surgery). This is discussed in greater detail in our chapter regarding donation complications. Many donors are economic providers for their family; thus, their death (or significant morbidity such as stroke) can add financial devastation to an emotional crisis. Families should be prepared in advance with a life insurance policy for the donor. This should be obtained before donation as there is a risk of higher premiums after donation.[6]

In the United States, the American Foundation for Donation and Transplantation and the Living Organ Donor Network (LODN) coordinate with participating transplant centers to offer life, health, and disability insurance to donors.[7] Donors can obtain information from LODN or the donor team social worker. The life insurance policy covers individuals from the time they leave their house to travel to the hospital for their donation and remains in effect for up to a year after any postdonation complications. The accidental death benefit is $500,000, and there is also a companion benefit for accidents affecting the support person who is traveling with the donor. The medical insurance policy covers $250,000 in expenses throughout the donor's lifetime. Mental health counseling has a $50,000 limit. If the donor is unable to work, the disability insurance policy provides income. Not all U.S. transplant centers participate in the LODN insurance plan because it requires the transplant center to pay a $550 enrollment fee for each donor as well as a $5,000 medical insurance deductible (amount paid by transplant center before the insurance policy begins paying for expenses). Nonetheless, donor candidates can purchase the insurance policy themselves regardless of transplant center participation.

We strongly advise all individuals to write a living will before they participate as donors. These documents are also known as advance directives, and they serve two important functions. First, the document is an official statement of an adult's health care treatment wishes in the event the person becomes cognitively impaired and cannot communicate with the medical team. In the document, the individual specifies what types of medical care are wanted and unwanted (e.g., artificial life support or cardiopulmonary resuscitation). The second function of the document is to inform the medical team who the adult has appointed as official decision maker for medical matters during times of critical illness. Often, individuals appoint their spouse, sibling, adult child, or best friend as surrogate. Both a primary and an alternate surrogate should be appointed in the event the primary is unavailable. Each state in the United States has its own unique laws regarding living wills, but in general they are very similar. The premise is that the surrogate decision maker (also known as durable power of attorney for health care) is ethically and legally bound to make decisions that correspond to the *patient's* wishes and values (even if this conflicts with the surrogate's own wishes and values). It is important to note that health care living wills do *not* give surrogates *any* decision-making powers with regard to property, bank accounts, mortgages, or other financial concerns. We suggest appointing surrogates who won't resist respecting and honoring written health care wishes; thus, it is important to discuss these concepts with family and friends beforehand. Once the living will is written, copies should be given to the surrogate(s) as well as the donor team and the donor's primary care physician. Living will templates are available at public libraries and on the Internet.[8]

Donor candidates who disregard the opinions or feelings of their spouse/ life partner raise concerns that need to be explored by donor teams. *Are the candidates in a state of tunnel vision that impacts their objectivity during their decision making? Do they understand that they are potentially putting their family relation- ships at risk of harm? Why would they take such risks and put their family under such stress?* Even when a spouse gives an organ to someone who is a genetic relative (or their marital partner), these donations can cause significant stress. As an example, eight married couples in Hong Kong were studied about the relationship consequences of living liver donation to their spouses.[9] The re- searchers anticipated that the interspouse donations would have increased the emotional bonds between the partners, but this was not always the case. In fact, while none of the eight spouses regretted their decision to donate, five of eight (63 percent) commented to the researchers that if they had the chance to live their life over again, they would marry a different person or not marry at all. Perhaps there was pressure for spousal donation (a culturally influenced assumption that the spouse would donate). The spouse may also be a caretaker in some way for his or her partner, and this might have added strain. These are speculations on our part, but clearly these donors did not become emotionally closer to their spouses as a result of donating an organ to them.

We asked our twenty-two Good Samaritan donors to describe to us the response of their families when they informed them of their desire to donate an organ. In general, most spouses/life partners were accepting even if they had fears about the donation process (seventeen of twenty-one). Two of twenty-one were not supportive, and another two were supportive but not happy about the idea. One donor did not have a spouse or life partner at the time of her decision to donate. Three donors took the approach of starting the donation process (the candidacy evaluation) before mentioning anything to their spouse/life partner. One had sketched out a plan but didn't realize it was impossible to accomplish: she theorized that she could complete the testing *and* donation surgery during the week while her husband was away on vacation—the donation would be a surprise when he returned home. She was surprised to find out how long the testing process can take. One donor countered her husband's arguments against donating by pointing out that he volunteered for risky activities himself: U.S. Special Forces military services. Seeing her valid point, he backed down. Another donor reported that her partner was fearful for her safety and would have preferred that she made a large monetary donation instead if she were financially able to. Even so, he supported her wish to give a kidney.

As we have shown, living donation can disrupt one's family even if the donation is to a spouse or close relative instead of a stranger. The marital stress can be significant.[10] We would like to see that relationships not be sacrificed in the name of Good Samaritan donation. We ask that donor candidates strongly consider *not* donating when their spouse/life partner has significant valid objections, such as those pertaining to financial strain. Another alternative to is come to an arrangement whereby both parties agree to disagree as a mutual condition in the setting of organ donation. In addition, it is ethically appropriate for candidates to consider the clinical needs of their own family members before they consider the clinical needs of strangers. Perhaps there is a history of organ failure requiring transplant in their own family, and thus there might be a future need for an interfamily organ donation. Jewish law supports the concept of adults being most responsible for those closest in relationship to them: "And the poor of his own household take precedence over the poor of his city."[11] An individual might have the clinical ability to be a Good Samaritan organ donor; however, in our view, there is no moral obligation to do so.

CHILDREN

Maturity is an important consideration when parents contemplate informing their children of living donation plans. The donor parent should reflect on three issues: 1) which child(ren) to inform, 2) when to tell the child, and 3) how to inform the child. Children of the same age may evidence a wide range of cognitive and emotional functioning, so their response to the concept of living donation can vary. Even a young child will likely wonder why a parent is making multiple trips to the hospital for "tests," and they should not be unnecessarily worried that their mother or father is sick. Children who have completed courses in science and biology in school will have a better grasp of the medical concept of organ donation than younger children who are learning to count and tie their shoes. Parents can use visual aids, such as anatomical models of a kidney or liver, or educational booklets available from the donor team social worker. An online company in Los Angeles sells colorful and humorous stuffed toys in the shape of anatomical body parts.[12] A coloring book about organ donation is also available for children ages six through nine.[13] Any medical information should be age appropriate so that it can be comprehended.

Altruism will likely be the harder concept to teach to children. Their experience in charity might be only dropping off used clothing and household goods at the Salvation Army, or maybe they have had more exposure: watching a parent donate blood, assisting with shoreline cleanup, or preparing food for the poor. Talking about Good Samaritan donation could cause a child to react with worry or fear that he or she is less valued than the stranger. This could occur in liver segment or lung lobe donations, as children are usually the recipients. Parents should provide reassurance to the child that while the gift is to an outsider, their child is family, and family creates special obligations—their child will never be forgotten, and his or her needs will always be addressed. Parents who want support during these discussions should seek the assistance of the donor team social worker who can be directly involved in conversations such as these with the child. In addition, the social worker can make arrangements for the child to meet other children of living donors and living donors themselves so that they can understand more about what the child and parent will be experiencing. Because Good Samaritan donation does not occur without also considering the needs of one's own family, it is important to have family, including young children, involved in the discussions.

· 24 ·

Organ Donation Surgery

*T*his chapter focuses on the general aspects of organ donor surgery, whereas the following chapter is devoted to the discussion of surgical complications. In this chapter, we discuss basic human anatomy, organ function, and surgery matters in order to help the reader gain an understanding of the impairments of those with organ failure as well as the "nuts and bolts" of living donor surgery. It's important to know about the human body and how it functions, as well as some of the changes that occur (e.g., scars) as a result of organ donation. As always, however, the donor surgical team is the best source of information because surgeons tailor the operation and aftercare according to the unique clinical features of the donor (e.g., body size, body shape, and medical and surgical history).

HISTORY OF ORGAN DONATION
AND TRANSPLANTATION

Before we explain (in lay terminology) the surgical techniques of the twenty-first century, it is important for readers to understand the history of donation and transplant. Both technologies have come a long way since 1954, when the first successful living donor transplant was performed. The surgeries, performed in Massachusetts, were profound because the donor–recipient pair was a set of identical twins; thus, their immune systems were also identical, allowing the recipient to tolerate his new kidney without any immunosuppressant medication. In fact, these medications did not exist at the time, so the only successful transplants that *could* occur were those between identical genetic pairs. In 1978, the first successful living pancreas donation occurred, and in 1987, the first successful living intestine transplant was performed. Two years later, the first successful living donor liver transplant occurred (adult to child), and a year after that, the first successful living lung transplant occurred. In 1994, a live individual simultaneously donated a kidney and a pancreas segment. In 1998, the first successful adult-to-adult living donor liver transplant occurred. By 2001, there were more living donors in the United States than deceased donors.

In the 1970s, general surgeons continued to use "open" techniques (large abdominal incisions) to perform surgery, while gynecologic surgeons were advancing their laparoscopic skills using small incisions filled with probes and camera equipment. By the 1980s, general surgeons were embracing laparoscopic technology for appendectomies, gallbladder removal, and hernia repair, and in 1995, they performed the first laparoscopic nephrectomy (kidney removal). With this advance, the risks to living donors were significantly reduced, as was the length of hospital stay. Currently, unless there is a complication, most donors who have a laparoscopic nephrectomy endure a hospital stay of less than forty-eight hours. Laparoscopic surgical techniques are now also widely used for living liver donation involving the left lateral segment from an adult to a child. While these techniques are lower risk because they involve smaller incisions, there is always the potential for an unforeseen event (e.g., hemorrhaging) that may require surgeons to convert from the laparoscopic technique to an open procedure. For this reason, donor candidates are always advised about this risk during the informed consent process.

KIDNEY DONATION (NEPHRECTOMY)

Most people are born with two kidneys, but some are born with only one (these people cannot be kidney donors). Even more rare, some people are born with three kidneys. The kidneys work as filters to purify the body of toxins and excess fluid. When the kidneys don't work properly, toxins build up and can be removed only by an artificial method called dialysis. Hemodialysis is a technique that takes several hours and involves removing blood from the body using a plastic tubing circuit and circulating it through special filters outside the body. The blood is then returned to the body. Patients usually receive hemodialysis three days per week. In peritoneal dialysis, a catheter fills the abdomen with dialysis solution. The abdominal cavity walls are lined with a membrane (peritoneum) that allows toxins and extra fluid to pass from the blood into the dialysis solution. The dextrose (sugar) in the solution pulls the toxins and extra fluid into the abdominal cavity and then leaves the body when the dialysis solution is drained. The process of draining and filling is called an exchange and takes about thirty to forty minutes. The period the dialysis solution is in the abdomen is called the dwell time. A common schedule is four exchanges a day, each with a dwell time of four to six hours. Both forms of dialysis are only temporary measures (and very burdensome) for patients who have kidney failure, leaving them often weak, tired, and nauseated. Their only cure for kidney disease is a kidney transplant.

There are three methods of kidney donation: open (longer recovery time and more painful), laparoscopic (least painful), and hand-assisted laparoscopic.[1] During an open procedure, a large incision (cut) is made in the abdomen, and the kidney is removed. During a laparoscopic procedure, several small incisions are made in the abdominal wall for insertion of video equipment and instruments that surgeons use to visualize, cut, and remove the kidney. Prior to removing the kidney, the surgeon wraps it with a plastic bag, and then the bagged kidney is pulled out of the abdomen through a short incision. Hand-assisted laparoscopic nephrectomy involves the surgeon placing his or her hand inside the body through one short incision while using smaller incisions for a video camera and instruments. The left kidney is most often removed because it has longer blood vessels and is not obstructed by the liver.

The open surgical procedure takes two to three hours, while the laparoscopic procedure takes longer (the surgeon is working in a smaller space with reduced visibility). While donors generally go home within forty-eight hours after laparoscopic surgery, they need about four weeks of recovery time without lifting (e.g., no carrying of children or grocery bags). Within two months after surgery, donors will receive a checkup (blood and urine testing) to evaluate their kidney function.

LIVER DONATION

The liver is the largest organ and it has two main functions: 1) converting food into energy and 2) removing alcohol and toxins from the blood. Liver failure can occur in many forms, such as a viral infection (hepatitis A, B, and C), liver cancer, alcohol or drug toxicity, and genetic defects, such as hemochromatosis (resulting in too much iron accumulating in the body). One of the most prominent symptoms of liver disease is jaundice (yellowing of the skin and "whites" of the eyes), which is caused by an accumulation of bilirubin in the blood.

The liver is a unique organ because of its ability to regenerate. It is for this reason that living liver donors can give a portion of their liver to a patient, and the donated portion grows into a full-size liver in about eight weeks. The remaining liver tissue in the donor will regenerate back to full size in approximately eight weeks as well.[2] While the liver does regenerate, a living liver donor can do so only one time. Repeat liver donations from the same donor are not possible. However, this does not prevent the liver donor from donating other organs. In our set of twenty-two living donors interviewed, we found several who wanted to be dual organ donors and one who did (kidney and liver). This donor reported no serious complications and great satisfaction with being a donor. She likened the experiences to giving the "perfect" gift to a friend and knowing how much they "love it." She is currently considering donating a lung lobe. As she explained, "I have been very lucky in my life. [I] have to give back."

Liver donation surgery can take five or more hours. When the donation involves an adult donor giving to an adult recipient, the donor receives a large vertical or upside-down T-shaped abdominal incision, and the liver is divided into two sections. If the donation involves an adult donating to a child, the surgery can often be performed using a laparoscopic technique. Depending on the size of the recipient, the donated portion of liver tissue may be smaller or larger (but not greater than 60 percent of the donor's liver volume). Several blood vessels (attached to the liver tissue) are also given to the recipient. Usually, the donor's gallbladder is also removed at the time of liver donation. The gallbladder is not needed for normal functioning. The donor's hospital stay is usually about one week, followed by at least four weeks of rest and recovery time at home. Strenuous activity and heavy lifting should be avoided for about six to eight weeks after donation.

Incisional staples are usually removed about ten days after surgery during a checkup. In addition, another follow-up visit will allow doctors to check the donor's liver with an ultrasound and laboratory tests to assess liver regeneration and functional status.

LUNG DONATION

The human lung is divided into five lobes: three on the right side and two on the left. Healthy lung functioning is essential in order to deliver oxygen to the brain. This is because in the smallest structures of the lungs, the alveoli, oxygen from the air we breathe diffuses into the bloodstream to all body tissues. Some lung transplants just replace the diseased lobes; however, recipients with cystic fibrosis (a disease that causes thick, sticky mucous) must have all their lung tissue removed when they are transplanted, or they risk infecting the donated tissue.

Living lung transplants are rare and unique because they require two living donors, each giving one lower lobe (right or left) to the recipient.[3]

The two donor lobes must be large enough to expand and fill the recipient's lung cavity (space), so generally only children and small adults receive living lung transplants. To remove the lobe, an incision is made on the side of the chest. The ribs are temporarily spread apart with a surgical tool so that the doctor can see the lung and deflate it. Blood vessels are then clamped and cut and the lobe removed. It is advised that the donor recover for six to twelve weeks before returning to employment. In the United States, the University of Southern California has the most experience with this procedure, and they conclude that living lung transplants are best for patients who are too sick to wait for a deceased donor transplant, but they are also suitable for those patients who would suffer significant clinical demise while waiting for deceased donor organs.[4]

OTHER DONATIONS

For information about partial intestine and partial pancreas donation surgeries, individuals should refer to the American Society of Transplantation.[5] Sometimes, when a partial pancreas is donated, the donor also donates a kidney at the same time. Intestinal donation usually involves about sixty inches of tissue from the middle section of the small intestine (the ileum). For information about bone marrow and stem cell donation procedures, individuals should contact the National Marrow Donor Program.[6]

SCARS

Because all living donations involve surgical incisions, all donors have scars on their skin. The size of the scar will vary according to the type of incision made (length, depth, and location), how it was sutured (closed), and how the donor's skin healed. Each person heals according to their own characteristics, such as genetics and age. The level of skin pigmentation (color) can also affect the scar's appearance. Because body image and cosmetic appearance are important to surgeons as well as patients, the concept of scarring is discussed with all potential living donors. This serves to provide information to the candidate as well as to educate the donor team about the candidate's fears, values and expectations.

There have been two published research studies on scarring and living donors. A study conducted in the Netherlands involved 125 kidney donors who had undergone either open (large incision) or laparoscopic (several small incisions) nephrectomy.[7] The donors completed a survey in which they ranked their satisfaction with their scar and the visual appearance of their scar. They also gave their scar a 1–10 rating (the larger the number the better). Donors from both groups gave their scars high ratings, indicating satisfaction with their body image and cosmetic appearance of the scar. In fact, the results were nearly the same for scars from either type of surgery (average laparoscopic rank score 8.5, average open rank score 8.6).

A study conducted in Canada involved 142 liver donors who had undergone right lobe donation.[8] The researchers used the same questionnaire as the Netherlands researchers and compared their results to them as well. Overall, they observed lower scores for the liver donors, and they suspect this could be due to the fact that the liver donation incision is generally much larger than that of open nephrectomy. Within the group of liver donors, they also reported that smokers were less satisfied with their score, but this is not surprising because smoking can negatively impact the healing of surgical scars (e.g., blood clots near the incision, loosened stitches, delayed healing, and infection). They also found that younger donors and nonwhite donors also had lower satisfaction scores. This could be due to younger people being more focused on their personal appearance and nonwhite donors having more pigmentation. This data would indicate that these groups might need more attention during predonation counseling about scarring.

In our group of twenty-two donors, only two reported numbness, tingling, or minor pain associated with their scar. One kidney donor developed a painful incisional hernia that required repair. Nearly all donors interviewed indicated they were proud to wear and even show off their scars to others. In fact, several donors were so proud of their scars that they sent us unsolicited photos of them. Feedback from our donors included describing their scars as "a badge of courage," "a badge of honor," and "the most beautiful mark on my body." Other donors reported, "I love it—it is a battle ribbon" and "My scars bring joy to my heart. They are there for a good reason." One donor went so far as to have a life-size tattoo of a kidney emblazoned on his back in the exact position where his donated kidney used to be.

If a surgical scar is thick, bulging, or tight, it can affect normal movement and cause discomfort. These matters should be reported to the donor team, as they can generally be corrected. Topical creams or gels to alter the appearance of scars should be used only with the approval of the donor team, as some of these products are ineffective and others can be harmful.

DONOR SURGERY TEAM

Living donation always involves two separate surgical teams: one for the donor and one for the recipient. Additionally, the donor and recipient are in separate (usually adjacent) operating rooms. Because all living donations require general anesthesia ("going to sleep" with medications and an airway tube down the throat), donors are also under the care of an anesthesiologist while in the operating room. This doctor monitors the donor's level of sedation breathing and blood pressure and assists with blood transfusions if needed. After surgery, the donor recovers under the care of medical and surgical teams in an intensive care unit, and then, as recovery progresses, the donor moves to a general ward until discharged home. Follow-up visits are essential to ensure the long-term safety and health of the living donors. In the United States, the costs for these visits are generally paid by the recipient's insurance policy or transplant center. It is important that donors report any medical or psychological complications (e.g., anxiety or depression) to the donor team so that they can respond to them and populate the living donor registry maintained by the United Network for Organ Sharing (UNOS). Such data are critical because they help UNOS monitor the safety profile of living donation as a technology as well as the safety profile of each U.S. transplant center that performs living donor surgeries.

As time evolves, surgical techniques and medical care evolve as well. This means that procedures and medications used with donors today might not be the same five years from now. As technology advances, donor surgeries will continue to be optimized for donor safety and welfare. As stated earlier, always consult with the donor team for the most up-to-date information about the surgical procedure and its associated hospitalization and aftercare.

· 25 ·

Complications

$\mathcal{A}$ discussion about living organ donation would be incomplete if it failed to include the topic of risks and complications. While we have presented several donor stories that show a spectrum of recovery times and experiences, we also want to inform the reader more fully about the latest clinical data on the safety of living donation. Our presentation is by no means a complete report of the scientific literature or world experience of living donation; rather, we have provided a snapshot of information for each type of donor surgery. Additionally, although we have cited clinical references that support the data presented, we remind the reader that technology is always evolving and that risks and statistics can change. In general, transplant centers that are more experienced at conducting donor surgeries should be the first choice for donation; however, we realize that some donor–recipient pairs may be limited in their options because of insurance restrictions that define the hospitals at which the surgeries can take place. Generally, Good Samaritan organ donations occur at high-volume transplant centers.

The risks of any surgery include infection, bleeding (possibly requiring a transfusion), pain, and complications from the anesthesia. These matters should be discussed with the donor team. Additionally, each specific type of organ donation has its own unique profile of risks. Some of this information is presented below; however, additional information is available from the donor team and the United Network for Organ Sharing (UNOS). In addition, it is advisable to speak with someone who has been a living donor so as to obtain firsthand experiential information. The transplant center social worker can arrange these meetings. Another mechanism is the International Association of Living Donors, which offers a free service of online donor mentors called Living Donor Buddies™.[1] It is also important to note that in the United States, if a living donor subsequently develops organ failure and needs a transplant, the individual will receive priority on the transplant waiting list. The exact details about this policy can be obtained from UNOS.[2]

KIDNEY DONATION

In 2009, researchers at the University of Minnesota published data from a large study (nearly 3,700 donors) that explored the safety of living kidney donation. They concluded that "survival and the risk of ESRD in carefully screened kidney donors appear to be similar to those in the general population."[3] Most of the donors in their study had an "excellent" quality of life after nephrectomy. Review of the U.S. registry data that contains mandatory reported information about donor complications finds that there were over 80,000 living kidney donors between April 1994 and March 1999, and they were followed for an average of 6.3 years by researchers in Baltimore.[4] They observed twenty-five donor deaths in the ninety-day period after surgery; however, this did not represent an increased mortality rate compared to the control group (nondonors). Surgical mortality from donation was 3.1 deaths per 10,000 donations. Mortality was higher in men and African Americans and those with high blood pressure (as compared to women, whites, Hispanics, and those without high blood pressure). Overall, long-term risk of death was no higher for living kidney donors than for the nondonors.

With regard to complications (morbidity) from nephrectomy, researchers have estimated that about 18 percent of donors experience a complication.[5] Men, older donors, and obese donors generally have higher complication rates than women, younger donors, and the nonobese. Women and older donors tend to remain longer in the hospital as they recover from their surgery. Of significant note, this study also found that hospitals that were low volume (fewer kidney donations than other hospitals) had more donors with complications and longer hospitalization periods as compared to higher-volume hospitals. Complications from donation can include injury to the gastrointestinal system (stomach and intestines), blood clots, and infection.

With regard to donor age, many transplant centers limit the maximum age of the living kidney donor; however, these cutoffs can vary widely from the middle fifties to the middle sixties. Current literature reports the oldest living kidney donor was eighty-four (and the recipient was eighty-three).[6] In contrast to the data from the study above, researchers in Kansas (2001–2005) looked at a smaller group of donors, comparing the complications of those older than age fifty to those of younger (the control group) and found complication rates in the two groups were nearly the same, 18 and 17 percent, respectively. For those receiving the organs, one-year transplant survival was 100 percent for those getting younger organs and 96 percent for those getting older organs. Overall, the researchers concluded that living kidney donation in donors older than fifty years of age "appears safe and demonstrates similar outcomes compared with the control cohort of patients younger than 50 years."[7] Another study, conducted in Baltimore on donors older than age sixty, found similar results and concluded that "laparoscopic donor nephrectomy may be performed safely in patients older than 60 years of age. There was no increase in complication rates or length of hospital stay."[8] What does this conflicting data mean if you are an older person considering being a donor? We suggest that older individuals optimize their health as much as possible (have few minor or no coexisting medical problems) and undergo surgery at a high-volume transplant center. This advice, of course, applies to all donor candidates.

UNOS advises potential kidney donors that the risks of kidney donation may include "high blood pressure (hypertension); large amounts of protein in the urine; hernia; organ impairment or failure that leads to the need for dialysis or transplantation."[9] In our experience interviewing sixteen kidney donors, most did very well during and after surgery, with generally minor complications (e.g., nausea and pain) or none at all. One donor did experience a life-threatening injury to her spleen requiring blood transfusions and conversion of the laparoscopic nephrectomy to an open surgery as well as spleen removal. Another experienced a painful incisional hernia that required repair and additional recovery time. Certainly, donors must remain vigilant after donation because giving one kidney means only one remains. If this kidney becomes damaged in the future (e.g., by disease or trauma like a car accident), there is the risk that dialysis or transplantation would be needed.

LIVER DONATION

Liver donation is a more complicated surgery than kidney donation; thus, the morbidity and mortality rates are higher. Additionally, these rates vary according to the type of donation performed (e.g., left lobe, right lobe, or left lateral segment) because of the amount of tissue removed and the risk of bleeding. The U.S. Department of Health and Human Services Advisory Committee on Organ Transplantation indicates that the risk of a complication from living liver donation is 15 to 30 percent (including a 0.2 percent risk of the donor needing a liver transplant) and estimates the risk of donor death at 0.2 percent (2 deaths in 1,000 donors).[10] Factors that increase the complication risk are older donor age, prolonged length of surgery, and right lobe donation.

Bile leaks are the most common complication. Most bile leaks get better without having another surgery, but they might require placement of tubes passing through the skin and into the liver to drain bile from the liver into a bag worn outside the body for a period of time. Other complications include small-bowel obstruction, infection, pain, incisional hernia (bulging at the scar), pleural effusion (excess fluid between the layers of pleural tissue in the chest), and biliary stricture (narrowing of the tube that moves bile from the liver to the small intestine).[11] In addition, there is the risk of organ impairment or failure that leads to the need for liver transplantation.

We interviewed five living liver donors, most of whom had a minor complications associated with donation. One donor had several months of postdonation nausea that severely impacted his quality of life until it abruptly vanished one day (to his great relief).

LUNG DONATION

As stated earlier, living lung donation requires two living donors to each contribute a lobe of one of their lungs; each lobe is then implanted into the recipient. Donors experience postoperative pain, but they are usually up and walking one to two days after donation and usually discharged in one to two weeks. However, it may take two to three months before normal activities can be resumed.

According to the American Society of Transplantation, approximately 4 percent of living lung donors experience a complication during surgery.[12] Less than 3 percent of live lung donors are readmitted to the hospital because of air in the chest cavity, heart rhythm problems, difficulty breathing, and so on. Complications lasting more than one year can include chronic incisional pain, difficulty breathing, inflammation around the heart, and nonproductive cough. Occasionally, donors have prolonged air leaks. Serious complications rarely occur but donors experience a 15 percent permanent decrease in vital capacity (the maximum amount of air a person can exhale after taking their deepest breath possible). Donors may be an increased risk of chest infection in the future, and if they develop lung disease, they will have less reserve. At this time, there have been no deaths due to living lung donation, but the risk always remains.

We interviewed one lung donor for our project. While he is ten years postdonation, he reports he is "nowhere where [he] used to be." He had a slow postoperative recovery that was complicated by an "allergic" reaction to a medication and problematic healing of his lung tissue, causing an air leak. While his vital capacity is reduced, he indicates that he detects this only when he hikes at high elevations. His scar still tingles and is painful at times, but he has no regrets and "would do it again in a heartbeat." More information about living lung donation can be obtained from the Second Wind Lung Transplant Association.[13]

WAKING UP AFTER SURGERY

In my (Dr. Bramstedt's) experience as a living donor advocate, the three most common complaints I hear about after a donor wakes up from surgery are pain, nausea, and vomiting. This is not abnormal, but donors should not hesitate to inform the medical team of the symptoms so that relief can be delivered. Pain is a normal part of surgery because of the cutting and body movements/anatomical shifting that were performed. Donors should not hesitate to ask for a consultation from a pain specialist ("pain consult") or other mechanisms, such as guided imagery, to help manage difficult symptoms. One of our twenty-two donors had an unusual experience in that her postoperative pain medication intravenous (IV) line stopped working, and she developed extreme pain. The fact that her IV needle had actually *fallen out* had gone undetected by the team taking care of her, and she was in fact not receiving any pain medication at all. On restoring medication delivery directly into her bloodstream, she obtained pain relief.

Nausea and vomiting can be caused by several factors, but sometimes these are side effects of the pain medications, and thus these medications may need to be changed. Medications to control nausea and vomiting can also be added. Additionally, donors shouldn't be too eager to consume steak or lasagna so soon after donation. It is best to follow the medical team's advice when they suggest ice chips or clear liquids. When the body is ready for solid food, only at that time will it be in the donor's best interest.

OTHER DONATIONS

As discussed earlier, individuals may also participate in other forms of living donation, namely, pancreas and intestine. For information about the risks of these procedures, contact UNOS[14] and the American Society for Transplantation.[15] For information about the risks of bone marrow/stem cell donation, contact the National Marrow Donor Program.[16]

PSYCHOLOGICAL OUTCOMES

The psychological impact of Good Samaritan donation has been studied by only a few research groups around the world. The most recent study, completed in

2010, concluded that Good Samaritan kidney donation had a "considerable positive impact" on the donor's psychological well-being and that their satisfaction with the donation experience was "very high."[17] Of the twenty-four donors who participated in the study, twenty-three indicated that they would still participate as a Good Samaritan kidney donor if they could rethink their choice (the twenty-fourth donor responded "maybe"). It should be noted that some individuals did report sleep disturbances after donation (it is unknown how long these persisted) and that some individuals were disappointed at the lack of contact between themselves and their recipient as well as other living donors (presumably for mentoring, camaraderie, and support). In another study of twelve Good Samaritan liver donors, the researchers reported that "none expressed regret about their decision to donate, and all volunteered the opinion that donation had improved their lives."[18] None of the twelve had a life-changing event after the donation, such as divorce, and one donor is writing a book about the donation experience.

In our experience interviewing twenty-two donors, we found similar results. All twenty-two were happy with their decision to donate and had no regrets about doing so. Only one donor was unsure if she would repeat the decision to donate, as she is currently fearful of health insurance discrimination. One donor suffered some depression as a result of a lengthy bout of post-donation nausea. Two donors expressed disappointment that they have not gotten to meet their recipients or have any contact with them. Another donor expressed "feeling bad" when his graft failed after transplant and his recipient returned to dialysis. He felt a connection to his kidney and the lack of success of the transplant and took it somewhat personally. Indeed, it is very important for donors to understand that recipient graft loss is a risk and that they, too, may feel this loss.

FINANCIAL ISSUES

While it is illegal to buy and sell organs in the United States (and most countries), federal law does allow donors to be reimbursed for expenses associated with the donation process (e.g., medical and surgical costs, meals, lodging, transportation, and lost wages). In the United States, there is no universal health care/national health insurance; therefore, the donor's medical and surgical fees related to the donation experience are paid for by the recipient's insurance policy. If there is a complication, the recipient's insurance policy covers the associated costs for a limited period of time, usually six to twelve months (varies by policy). This said, if a donor experienced a late or lengthy complication, there is the very real risk of having expenses that would not be paid by the recipient's insurance policy. It is for this reason that we strongly recommend that donors have their own personal health insurance to fill this gap and protect their clinical and financial welfare.

Other financial matters to consider include time away from work and child care expenses. Many employed donors have "sick time" or "vacation time" benefits that they use so that their paychecks remain uninterrupted. In the United States, federal employees are entitled to use seven days of paid leave each calendar year to serve as a bone marrow donor and up to thirty days of paid leave each calendar year for organ donation.[19] If more time is needed, loss of pay can result. Some employers have avoided this dilemma by allowing coworkers to donate paid time to the organ donor. The transplant center social worker can advise potential donors about the available state, federal, and charitable benefits to compensate for lost income and child care.

In the United States, the recipient is permitted to reimburse the donor for costs directly associated with the donation. In addition, the National Living Donor Assistance Center provides financial aid.[20] For those who apply for help, most (88 percent) are approved for funding (there are income and citizenship restrictions). Approved donors receive an American Express® Controlled Value Card (CVC) to purchase airfare, gas, rental cars, hotel rooms, food, and other incidental expenses, such as parking. Funds are added or removed to the CVC as needed by program staff. Additionally, most transplant centers have their own private assistance funds that can help donors with some of their financial needs. Another source of funding for lost wages and living expenses of kidney donors is the Heal With Love Foundation.[21] For expenses that remain unreimbursed, these may be tax deductible. A certified public accountant can provide more information on tax codes and tax deductions.

ORGAN STEWARDSHIP—HOW YOU CAN HELP

If you are considering participating as a living donor, it is critical to remember that you are entering surgery as a *healthy* person who does not *need* any surgery at all (a paradox). It is very important that you arrive at the operating room in optimal medical condition and exit it the same way. Being a good steward of your body beforehand is recommended (e.g., discontinue smoking and stay within the target weight/body mass index range suggested by the transplant center). Additionally, transplant centers often have other, more specific advice, such as discontinuation of birth control pills prior to donation (to reduce the risk of stroke). Consult with your transplant center about these optimization measures in order to promote your safety and welfare.

VII

LIFE AFTER
ORGAN DONATION

· 26 ·

Kevin: Canada's First
Good Samaritan

$\mathcal{A}$s the eleventh of thirteen children, Kevin knows what it means to share. His smile-shaped abdominal scar is evidence of that—in 2005 he shared his liver with a ten-year-old boy he has never met.[1] And because he was Canada's first Good Samaritan liver donor, the news made headlines.[2] But more important, it spawned sixteen more Good Samaritan liver donations at Toronto General Hospital.[3]

As a child, Kevin had many career aspirations: doctor, carpenter, department store manager, and police officer. For a time, he worked at his father's travel agency. He also spent five years in the army reserves and earned a second-degree black belt in karate. He eventually found his niche in supervision and productivity improvement for Kraft in the food industry, and this is where he has worked for the past twenty-seven years. It's really no surprise that there is a connection between his job and his liver donation because both focus on the same thing: enhancement, making something better. By giving his left lateral liver segment to a child with a urea cycle enzyme deficiency, the boy no longer suffers from a buildup of toxic ammonia in his blood, and his body can metabolize protein normally (essential for proper growth and brain functioning).

In the summer of 2004, the path of a new life for this child began. The boy's liver was not working, and neither was Kevin's car. Oddly, this brought the two of them together. While Kevin was familiar with organ transplantation because he had known a few people who had received kidney transplants, he had never considered being a living organ donor until he found himself captive in the waiting room of an auto repair shop, reading an article about the topic in a magazine. "I knew people really needed the help and there was an organ shortage."[4] He knew he could make a difference. For Kevin, his thought process was "Are you just going think about it, or are you actually going do something about it? . . . so I thought I'm *going* do something about it."[5] The stories he read in the magazine stirred up his compassion, and he felt that someone was depending on him to help.

Similar to many of the other Good Samaritan donors we interviewed, Kevin had a very difficult time giving his liver tissue to a stranger. In Canada, this had never been done before, so the hospitals he approached were very nervous about the idea. *Was Kevin crazy? Why would a healthy man with a stable marriage and career want to do this?* Kevin wondered why the hospitals were so concerned and why they seemed to overcomplicate the process. According to Kevin, "I've had a pretty good life and been blessed in so many ways. I have nothing to complain about. It's just a nice thing to do because somebody needs it. . . . I am capable and I am willing."[6] He also had no desire to choose or meet his organ recipient. All he wanted to do was help.

But Kevin's statements alone were not convincing. Only one transplant hospital was willing to evaluate him. The others turned down his organ offer. What ensued was a nine-month journey of tests and consultations to ensure that he was medically and psychologically fit and that his motives were ethically appropriate. In addition to the clinical assessments led by Dr. Gary Levy and Dr. Ian McGilvray, he was interviewed by a social worker, a clinical ethicist (twice), two psychiatrists, and a donor advocate (this role is discussed in detail in chapter 22). Kevin was able to rationally explain to these individuals why he opted for liver donation instead of kidney donation: he wanted to reserve kidney donation in case a relative needed it because there was a history of kidney disease in his family. In addition, he knew that for those who have kidney disease, they at least have dialysis as an option, whereas those with liver failure have no bridging option and need a lifesaving liver transplant. His logic was indisputable. He feels the role of the ethicist was very helpful to the assessment process because this person was able to reflect on the contextual features of the case, such as his religious values (Anglican) and his history of prosocial behavior, such as blood donation, volunteer work, and marrow donor registration. The ethicist was able to pull the package of data together to present a man with altruistic motivations.

Kevin's donation was somewhat unique because he and his recipient were located at two different hospitals: one for adults (Toronto General Hospital) and one for children (The Hospital for Sick Children). When Kevin's liver tissue was removed, it was transported across the street to his awaiting recipient in a pediatric operating room. He vividly remembers lying down on the operating table and thinking that across the street a child was doing the same. As if sending the child a telepathic message, Kevin thought, "Don't worry, sweetheart. Part of me is coming to help. I'm committed. I didn't give up. I'm here."[7]

Kevin was hospitalized for one week, and nine weeks later he was back at work. It has been five years since his donation, and Kevin continues to feel well. For his safety, the hospital will follow him clinically for at least ten years. He has experienced no medical or psychological complications but did incur several thousand dollars in unreimbursed expenses for travel, meals, and lodging associated with his trips to the hospital for assessment and surgery. At the time, Canada did not have provisions for reimbursing these types of expenses, but now the provinces have special programs that give donor's financial assistance.[8]

Kevin is glad he participated as a living donor and has no regrets, even though he experienced significant financial costs. His family supported his decision, and he states he would do it again if he had the opportunity to retrace his steps. In fact, recently he tried to become an anonymous kidney donor but was declined during the testing process because of new-onset type 2 diabetes. Even the fact that he has never met his recipient has not dulled his enthusiasm. A year after the donation, he received a thank-you letter from the child's parents. Below is an extract from their letter, which was read during a hospital press conference:

> Hope for us came in the form of an angel-donor named Kevin who was willing to risk an operation which he did not need so that our child could begin to live a carefree and normal life. For the first time, our child is now able to eat meat, fish, dairy, bread & pasta and now enjoys new-found favorite foods such as pancakes & McDonald's Happy Meals, making new friends and playing without the need to take so many medications so often! What freedom! What joy!
>
> We are so profoundly grateful to you, Kevin, and your family, for fearlessly and with great compassion giving our child hope and the possibility of a future. How can we explain to you what it is like not to have a worry every minute of the day that your child could suffer irreversible brain damage or even die?
>
> Thank you Kevin, thank you Kevin's family for giving us a part of yourselves which we will treasure, cherish and nurture every day as we watch our child grow into adulthood because of your precious Gift of Life.

People in need of an organ will tell you that people like Kevin are "angels." Maybe he is. He never worried about his surgery and never had any doubts about the appropriateness about what he was doing. For Kevin, Good Samaritan donation was just a "nice" thing to do, and it saved a life.[9]

· 27 ·

Claude: Ready to Rescue

$\mathcal{I}$magine a dark night, with fog lurking above the waterline of a small river in a remote land. Think of a place as far away as your brain will allow. Swimming stealthily through the muddy water is a man wearing a wetsuit and camouflage face paint. As he crawls through the reeds up the riverbank, he checks his global positioning satellite device to resume navigation. He hasn't slept or eaten in twelve hours, but he is as fresh as the morning sun. He is on a mission. If you are a hostage, you are on Claude's radar. If you are a terrorist, be very afraid. Claude has been trained as a paracommando. He can parachute out of airplanes, hike rough terrain, rappel ice crevices, open locks, and rescue captives. He will lay his life on the line for you. He will even give a piece of his liver. That's what he did in 2005.[1]

Claude's training as a Belgian armed forces paracommando rendered him a capable lifesaver, but there was nothing about living organ donation in his training manual or curriculum. And, as Claude found out, just as it is challenging to rescue captives, it can also be challenging to donate a liver segment. As much as he wanted to give it away to a stranger, finding a receptive transplant hospital was very difficult.[2] But the story goes back farther than that, as Claude had also attempted to be a bone marrow donor to his niece, but he was not an immunological match. When a match was finally found, she died hours before the marrow transplant. While Claude is a firm believer that death is very much a part of life, he still wanted to try to save a life, even if he could not save his relative.

Talking to Claude, it is evident that this man is fearless. Not that this is surprising for a man who is known for jumping out of airplanes and hiking frozen regions with weapons in tow. Claude had more than one near-death experience in his lifetime, including surviving the rupture of a brain aneurysm in 2001. He spent a month in the hospital recuperating, yet that experience did not scare him away from the clinical setting. It is ironic to spend a month, critically ill in a hospital, and then *voluntarily* return to an operating room at a later date for an unneeded surgery: liver donation.

This irony, of course, was on the minds of the clinicians who received his donation request. Doctors repeatedly asked him, "Why do you want to do this?" In Europe, Good Samaritan donation was nearly nonexistent. In fact, the only other case was a Good Samaritan kidney donation in Germany in 1966.[3] That case did result in a temporary increase in living donations; however, Germany later banned Good Samaritan organ donation because of fears of organ trafficking. The offer of liver donation was very unconventional and made many hospitals nervous. He searched the Internet in an attempt to find a hospital what would accept his organ donation. Even hospitals in the United States declined his offer. Claude finally sought help from the Euroliver Foundation,[4] which referred him to a liver surgeon at the Saint-Luc University Clinics in Brussels. This surgeon, Jean-Bernard Otte, was a cofounder of the Euroliver Foundation, and he was able to initiate Claude's medical and psychosocial consultations.

Just like our other donors, Claude was evaluated by a psychiatrist as well as the usual medical doctors and surgeons. He was even interviewed by the hospital's ethics committee. What is unusual in this case is that Claude had to pay for all these expenses himself (e.g., laboratory and screening tests and physician consultations). Nonetheless, he was not deterred. At fifty-one years of age, Claude was looking to help someone in need and looking for a challenge in life. Living donation met his criteria. He worried that his wife, however, would not be as excited as he was about the idea. Thinking that she might react unfavorably to the concept, Claude didn't tell her about his plan until he had been accepted as a donor by the hospital. To his surprise, she supported him (even though she was fearful of doctors and hospitals). His daughter, a student studying to be an anesthesiologist, was also supportive.

Claude's recipient was a twelve-year-old boy with Alagille syndrome. This is a genetic disorder in which a person has fewer than the normal number of small bile ducts inside the liver. The ducts drain bile from the liver into the gallbladder, so when there is a small number of them, bile builds up inside the liver, causing liver damage and jaundice (yellowing of the skin and the whites of the eyes). Severe itching and small deposits of fat under the surface of the skin are also common complications. The only cure for this anatomical defect is a liver transplant, giving the patient new liver tissue that has genetic programming for the appropriate number of small bile ducts. Sometimes there are also facial deformities, such as deep-set eyes; a straight nose; a prominent, pointed chin; and a prominent, wide forehead. These, of course, are not remedied with a liver transplant, but they are not life-threatening maladies. The child had been waiting for a deceased donor liver transplant for more than two years when Claude's gift of a left liver segment came his way. Because liver tissue regenerates, Claude's remaining tissue was restored to a full-size liver, and the 270-gram segment given to the child grew into a full size liver as well.

Claude hopes that someday he will get to meet the child who is currently seventeen years old. If the two eventually meet, it will be with the consent of the recipient, as currently there is still a confidentiality agreement in force (written prior to the donation as a condition of the ethics committee to allow the surgery to go forward). For now, Claude cherishes the thank-you letter the boy's mother sent him after the surgery as well as the letter the boy sent him five years later (translated from French to English and reprinted with permission of the donor):

> Dear Friend,
> Five years have gone by since the transplant. During these last years I grew up a lot. I love to go to school. I am very content to have succeeded each year. I love to learn new things and make new buddies.
> Currently, I am visiting Brussels for the routine checkup. The results of the biopsy are good and that's what makes me happy.
> I am you and will always be grateful for the gift you gave me. Thanks to you I can lead a normal life: go to school, play with my buddies, and simply enjoy life.
> I want to thank you, with my family, again with all my heart for the sacrifice that you made for me.
> I hope that all is well with you. I would be pleased to hear your news. Are you doing good?
> [signed] A very grateful friend

Claude was born the middle of five children. His father was a clerk and his mother a teacher, but his role model in life was his uncle, a doctor. Like other donors we interviewed, Claude had a history of service work in his family, and he could have modeled some of their behavior when he did service efforts such as translation activities, military enlistment, enrollment on the bone marrow registry, and liver donation. Additionally, his motivation for liver donation was so altruistically pure that the offer of a mere "1 Euro"[5] would have stopped him in his tracks. He would not let anything contaminate the pure generosity of his gift, and he firmly declares that he does not want to be considered a hero.

Claude's life continues to be filled with exciting moments because he now works as a volunteer firefighter and ambulance worker. His liver donation has not slowed him down one bit. On a quiet day, you'll find him basking in his home with the windows wide open or possibly in his studio doing woodworking projects. He has no regrets about donating and would repeat his decision if given the opportunity. He hoped his gift, the first Good Samaritan liver donation in Europe, would have paved the way for more donations, but this has not happened. This is his only disappointment. Claude knows the benefits of living donor transplantation and wants others to experience them too.

· 28 ·

The Organ Recipient:
Ethical Considerations

$\mathscr{B}$ecause Good Samaritan organ donation is actually a two-part process (do-nation and transplantation), it is difficult if not impossible to *not* look beyond the donation to the transplant. But because what happens in the transplant setting is separate from the donor and a private matter for the recipient, do-nor candidates are always counseled that there is the possibility that they may never learn the identity of the recipient of the organ, never meet him or her, and never even get a thank-you letter. Donor candidates are warned that there may be a black hole of information and gratitude and that this could be a source of distress. Usually, this warning does not dissuade candidates from pursuing donation, as they desire to donate not for the purpose of recognition but from a helping motivation that requires nothing in return.

PRIVACY

Some transplant hospitals are so concerned about maintaining the privacy of the organ recipient and donor that they go to great lengths to keep their identities secret as well as their locations during hospitalization. For example, some hospitals assign alias names to their donors and recipients. Sometimes, they are given rooms on different floors of the hospital. Even these measures are occasionally not enough to prevent their identities from being revealed. At least one of the donors we interviewed ended up meeting his intended recipi-ent at the laboratory where they both went for blood tests.[1] A donor in San Diego met her intended recipient in the hospital elevator as both were called for surgical admission.[2] There are also cases of family members of the donor and recipient meeting each other in communal waiting rooms. Because both the donor and recipient are considered patients, their medical information and privacy are protected under U.S. law. Medical teams generally cannot share personal information between the two parties unless there is mutual consent. The only exception is medical information that is critical to the transplant.

As we discussed earlier, most of our Good Samaritan organ donors had no desire to choose their organ recipients or even meet them postoperatively. Only one donor indicated that meeting the recipient was critical to the donation experience. This kidney donor wanted to personally see the benefit that the patient received in order to make the donation experience "more real."[3] Another donor admitted that after donating, she developed an intense curiosity about her organ recipient and has been trying to determine his or her identity using the Internet.[4] Hospitals generally broach the subject of donor–recipient contact with each member of the pair before their surgeries to ask them their preference about meeting each other. The decision is then documented in the medical record. It's important to note that the donation and transplant experience can have profound impacts such that individuals who originally (presurgery) wanted to maintain anonymity might ultimately opt for meeting the other half of their pair. After surgery, if one or both of the parties decide they want to meet, a request is made to the hospital transplant center, and their personnel make a careful approach to the individual. The approach must be delicate because the individual may have indicated prior a desire not to meet the other party, or he or she may be experiencing surgical or other complications—they may have feelings of anger, frustration, depression, grief, and so on.

If the two parties do consent to meet, hospitals often require a "cooling-off" period. This is a period that ranges between several weeks to several months (there is no standard) and that is designed to give both parties time to return to their baseline medically and psychologically. The location of the meeting is sometimes a neutral place, like a park or restaurant, so that both parties maintain their privacy in terms of their home and family life. For some, the meeting can be a quiet conversation between just the two of them. For others, it is planned as a spectacular event with balloons, flowers, and food galore.

Sometimes, there is no meeting of the pair, but the donor receives a thank-you card or letter from the recipient. In other cases, there is no contact at all, not even a note of thanks. The latter can be a shock or discouraging to some donors. Most of the Good Samaritan donors we interviewed have met their recipients in person (sixteen of twenty-two). Of the six who did not, one received a thank-you letter from the family of his pediatric recipient, one received a thank-you letter from the family of his pediatric recipient shortly after donation as well as a thank-you letter from the child five years later, and another had short term email contact with her recipient but then lost contact when her computer malfunctioned and she irretrievably lost the recipient's email address.

For the few of our donors who have not met their recipient, this has not been without effect on them. As indicated, one donor, while not concerned with meeting the recipient, desperately wants to discover his or her identity and is using the Internet in an attempt to do so.[5] Another donor felt that she was given false hope by the transplant center that she would likely eventually meet her organ recipient. To date, this has not happened, and she is disappointed but has been able to "put the idea to rest."[6] One donor knew explicitly that he would not get to meet his recipient because this was a condition to the donation's being allowed to occur.[7] Nonetheless, he feels that he should, at a minimum, be privy to medical and quality-of-life updates about the clinical status of his organ recipient.

In the setting of donations to pediatric recipients, it is understandable why some parents might want to maintain their privacy and that of their child. The child has been suffering a life-threatening illness and may not understand a stranger coming into his or her life. Even though the organ gift is valuable and appreciated, it may overwhelm the child and family. These reasons sometimes result in families (and/or the child) writing thank-you letters to their donors instead of pursuing face-to-face contact. Whatever the reasons and situations, donors should respect the privacy of their recipients. Similarly, recipients should respect the privacy of donors who wish to remain anonymous.

THANK-YOU GIFTS

If a recipient offers a thank-you gift to the donor, this must be a moderate form of appreciation and gratitude, not payment for the organ. (Organ vending is not only unethical but also illegal in the United States and most countries.) If the gift seems unusually grand, the donor should ask him- or herself, "How would I feel if the public knew I received this gift? How would the United Network for Organ Sharing feel about a donor receiving a gift of this nature?" If the answers pose ethical discomfort, this is a sign the gift is inappropriate. Organ recipients can pay their donors' medical and surgical costs, transportation, housing, meals, child care expenses, and lost wages associated with the donation process, but recipients must never pay a fee for the organ itself. Organs are gifts. They are donations. They have no price tag. Check any U.S. hospital bill—the patient is never charged for the organ itself.

The National Kidney Foundation has created a website for organ recipients who are having difficulty finding suitable thank-you gifts for their living donors.[8] At this website, organ recipients post their ideas to share them with the transplant community. Dozens of ideas are suggested, including kidney-shaped chocolates, inexpensive kidney-shaped jewelry, T-shirts, coffee mugs, photo albums and memorial books, and flower bouquets. If an organ recipient felt strongly about making a large financial donation, this should not be given to the organ donor; rather, it should be given to a charitable organization. Ethically, it would not be unreasonable for the organ donor to participate in selecting the charity. Potential ideas include organizations that provide grants to donors for costs associated with donation, organizations that conduct research on organ failure and transplantation, and organizations that promote organ donation awareness. If a living donor is offered payment for his or her organ, this should be rejected and the recipient advised that such payments are illegal. The donor should suggest other mechanisms of thank-you, such as those suggested above. The organ recipient may feel that a deep debt needs repayment; however, the donor should provide reassurance that no repayment is needed. Verbal expressions of gratitude are enough for the altruist. When the recipient is compliant with medical advice and medication management (organ stewardship), this is also very much appreciated by donors.

BONDING

Some living donors develop strong bonds with their organ recipients. We confirmed this when we interviewed our Good Samaritan donors. Fred was still asleep in his hospital bed when his kidney recipient came by to see him.[9] Her room was only a few doors away from his. She did not want to disturb him, so she left a note on his pillow informing him, "Your kidney visited."[10] They had a face-to-face meeting in the hospital not long after that, and they continue to get together at an annual bonfire event at Fred's home. Fred refers to his recipient as "my kidney caretaker"[11] and states she will always have a place in his life. In fact, when they are together, he likes it when she stands on his left side because he gave her his left kidney. He refers to his recipient as "a very warm thought."[12]

Chad met his kidney recipient ten days after donation. Unfortunately, she contracted a viral infection soon after she was discharged from the hospital and had to be readmitted for further care. Chad went to the hospital to meet her. There, he also met her husband and her mother. Chad's Good Samaritan donation was both a lifesaver and a life changer for the recipient. After her transplant, she quit her job in California and returned to her home country, Australia, where she enrolled in medical school. She is intending to pursue transplant medicine as a career. Chad and his recipient converse via email and Facebook, and his daughter spent three months visiting her "Down Under."

One of our donors bonded with both her recipient as well as the recipient's wife.[13] On occasion during phone calls with the recipient's wife, the donor noticed her to be crying. During these calls, she would confide to the donor that the recipient had been emotionally abusive. After observing a pattern of this abuse, the donor called the recipient and angrily informed him that his behavior was inappropriate and needed to stop. She also told him that if she could, she would take out his kidney and give it to someone else. This seemed to shake up the recipient, and he improved his behavior with his spouse. The donor cries when she thinks of the times she spent with her recipient, as he is now deceased. During the nearly ten years he lived with her kidney, they shared birthdays and Christmas holidays together. Her recipient loved cherries, so she would bring him a cherry pie or cherry ice cream every time she went to visit. His wife liked bagels, so she would bring a gift of bagels and cream cheese for her. She also organized a fund-raiser when the recipient's spouse lost her job. When asked if she feels her relationship with them was extremely close, the donor told us, "Oh yeah."[14]

Max told us there is "no doubt" there is a bond between him and the recipient of his kidney.[15] In fact, he feels like he has a new family member. Max met his recipient while both were recovering in the hospital. He was still a little groggy from the anesthetic, but he remembers her bright smile. He describes talking with her as a "joyful experience."[16] A year after the donation, when the recipient was interviewed by a local television station, she stated, "You just know that it's instant friendship and it's everlasting."[17] Laura had been a healthy college student who suddenly developed life-threatening kidney failure due to a rare autoimmune disease called Wegener's granulomatosis. Max's gift saved her life and allowed her to graduate from school.

Bonding can be a good thing, but we also caution that any time there is even a hint of pathological behavior, such as stalking, this should be reported to the transplant hospital and police immediately. In addition, if there are attempts at financial extortion, this should also be reported to law enforcement personnel and the living donor advocate.

ILLNESS AND DEATH

While organ transplants are generally lifesaving, they do not grant their recipients immortality. According to the Department of Health and Human Services, five- and ten-year survival rates for recipients of living kidneys are 98.9 and 79.9 percent, respectively.[18] The five- and ten-year survival rates for living liver recipients are 91.7 and 67.9 percent, respectively.[19] Because the donor organ is considered foreign, it will be rejected by the recipient's body unless the recipient takes powerful antirejection medications called immunosuppressants. These medications can cause numerous side effects, such as nausea, vomiting, headaches, facial hair, facial swelling, and mood swings. Some of these problems can be fixed by switching to a different medication or adjusting the dosage. The most notable and unavoidable problem with immunosuppressants is that the recipient, consequently, has a weakened immune system and is prone to infection. Infections such as colds or flu can impact a transplant patient so severely that hospitalization is required.

Another problem for organ recipients is cancer. Organ transplant recipients have a fifty- to one-hundred-fold fold higher incidence of squamous cell cancer compared to nontransplant patients.[20] These are malignant cancers that affect the squamous cell layer of various areas of the body, such as the skin, lips, mouth, esophagus, urinary bladder, prostate, lungs, vagina, and cervix. Transplant recipients are also at increased risk of developing melanoma either from sun exposure (ultraviolet radiation) or from donor-transmitted disease.[21] Melanoma is a form of skin cancer originating from the skin's pigment cells.

Transplant recipients can have a rough road. Even if they don't encounter problems with infections or cancer, they can experience recurrence of the disease that caused their native (original) organ failure. For example, patients who undergo transplantation due to liver failure caused by hepatitis B or hepatitis C often get recurrence of the virus months to years later.[22] Autoimmune organ failure, when the body mistakenly attacks itself, can also recur in the patient, affecting the new organ. For example, while the three main types of autoimmune liver disease can all be treated with liver transplant, there is always the risk of recurrence. The recurrence risk for primary sclerosing cholangitis (swelling, scarring, and destruction of the bile ducts inside and outside the liver) is 10 to 27 percent,[23] the recurrence rate for autoimmune hepatitis (liver inflammation) is 50 percent after ten years,[24] and the recurrence rate for primary biliary cirrhosis (irritation and swelling of the bile ducts of the liver) can be as high as 50 percent.[25] All three have the potential to cause organ failure and the need for retransplant. Autoimmune kidney disease also sometimes recurs after kidney transplantation.[26]

Another unfortunate situation of recipient illness is that which is caused by noncompliance, which can take many forms. Sometimes, patients fail to adhere to the transplant team's requirement for a special diet and weight control. Sometimes, they don't take their medications as prescribed. This can be due to many factors, ranging from complacency to side effect intolerance to lack of medication access resulting from financial difficulties. Medical evidence assures us that failure to follow the advice of the transplant team will guarantee organ failure. This is why the screening process that selects patients as organ transplant candidates is so rigorous. Knowing that organs are scarce gifts and that living donors put their lives on the line to save others, transplant teams are very careful to thoroughly screen for transplant candidates who have the greatest chance at success. In medical ethics terms, this is called "capacity to benefit." Nonetheless, even careful screening can fail to disqualify all those who might be noncompliant after transplant. Teams look for a history of pre-transplant compliance, a motivated attitude (truly desiring a transplant rather than ambivalence), the will to live, the absence of addiction and behavioral problems, and a strong psychosocial support system (including financial stability). In the setting of pediatric transplants, noncompliance has been shown to be a major barrier to success—especially for adolescents. They sometimes can't resist the temptation to stop their medications when unsightly side effects like acne, inappropriate facial hair, and facial swelling appear. And when they feel great, the attitude of being cured can also be a tempting lure to cease or reduce their medication dosing.[27]

When donors become aware of their recipient's illness, this can be stressful for them. Three of our twenty-two Good Samaritan donors have experienced the death of their organ recipient. Ken, an artist and the first person in the world to give a liver lobe to an adult stranger, has experienced the emotional pain of his recipient's illness and passing.[28] Deborah was thirty-nine years old when they accidentally met in the hospital waiting room. Deborah had contracted an infection after a blood transfusion, and the virus was destroying her liver. Ken had heard her father's pleas for a liver donation on television and immediately responded to the need. Thanks to Ken, Deborah lived an additional nine years and was able to see her daughter marry. She was also able to spend time with her father before he passed away. In 2008, Deborah died of complications from kidney failure. This was devastating for Ken.[29] While she eventually lost her life, Ken came to realize how much life she was able to experience in the nine extra years she was given because of the transplant. Ken has no regrets about donating the right lobe of his liver and says he would "do it again in a second. You don't know what you're missing!"[30]

Curt, also a liver lobe donor to an adult, experienced a similar loss, but much sooner.[31] His organ recipient died of pneumonia four months after transplant. They had kept in touch after surgery, and he bonded with him and his family, even though they were from different religious and cultural backgrounds. The funeral was attended by nearly 500 people, and Curt gave the eulogy. After the funeral, as a gesture of appreciation and memorialization, the family gave Curt the pall, which had covered the coffin. As with Ken, Curt described himself as being "devastated" at the loss of his recipient. The transplant was supposed to have saved him from his prior years of sickness, and yet he experienced only four months of health. Curt felt a myriad of emotions during the time of this loss, but looking back he has no regrets and would repeat his donation decision if he had the chance.

Dave, a Good Samaritan lung lobe donor, is unique in that he witnessed his recipient undergo two transplants: one from himself in 2000 and another transplant (from a deceased donor) in 2008.[32] Dave's recipient was Matthew, a scrawny teenage surfer who was able to return to the waves following his living donor transplant. He was also able to travel to exotic places like Fiji and experience other cultures. This young man was profoundly impacted by life extension and the miracle of transplant, so much so that he created the Big Worm's CF Foundation to help other children impacted by cystic fibrosis. Through Dave's gift of a lung lobe, there were the benefits of improved quality of life, employment, travel and more surfing for Matthew. Even now, the foundation continues to help improve the quality of life of hospitalized cystic fibrosis patients by providing them with toys, electronics, and other gifts. Matthew's funeral was held at sea, his favorite place. A surfboard topped with fresh flowers was sent adrift, and his ashes were scattered in the water. More than one hundred surfers sat on their boards in the California ocean in remembrance of this vibrant and compassionate young man. Matthew's donor has no regrets about the donation, and, in fact, he believes that it was what God wanted him to do for this boy. Dave values the fact that he got to talk to the boy about his belief in God and considers it his opportunity to witness to him about his spirituality and faith. He has peace knowing that he did God's will by participating as Matthew's donor.[33]

Isaiah was another teenager whose life was changed by a Good Samaritan donor. Garrett, an attorney in Ohio, gave him one of his kidneys in 2005.[34] Unfortunately, he contracted BK virus (named after the initials of the patient first observed with this condition) and subsequently lost his graft and returned to dialysis. Garrett was familiar with loss, having experienced the death of his first wife to cancer. Nonetheless, the graft loss was a profound event that saddened him. Garrett had come to the aid of this autistic child who also had a host of other problems, including bone deformities, a heart murmur, and a small bladder. His kidney donation had enabled the child to be freed from the burdens of dialysis and attain honor roll status as well as a part-time job. He also was able to return to participating in sports activities with his peers. Early on, just days after the transplant, the child's mother put it all in perspective when she referred to Garrett as her "angel" and said, "Whether this kidney lasts a week, a month, a year, he [Garrett] will always be in my heart."[35]

For those donors who have never had any contact with their organ recipients (or their families) there is a black hole of information in terms of their clinical status. Are the recipients dead or alive? Healthy or ill? For the emotional health of the donor, we suggest that donor teams consider this concept very early in the transplant process. In fact, we think that it would be ethically appropriate for donor teams to notify donors of their recipient's death so that they can grieve the loss of their organ gift and find closure. We think the best way to accomplish this is to ask donors during the informed consent process if they want this information (should it become available to the hospital) and a record of their answer to be placed in their medical chart. If the recipient dies, the date of death would be given to the consenting donor. Details about the circumstances associated with the death should remain confidential unless the recipient's family consents to such information disclosure (e.g., cause of death and age of patient). It is foreseeable that some families might consent to allow the donor to be present at the funeral; however, donors should not expect this and should respect the privacy of the recipient's family.

• 29 •

Life after Donation

$\mathscr{T}$he life of an organ donor will never be the same after donation. Psychologically, the donor will have experienced a significant emotional event, namely, saving the life of another human. Physically, the body will be changed (even if there are no medical complications). As discussed earlier, there can be indirect benefits to the donor, and these do not mar the altruistic nature of the donation. These side effects were not the ultimate goal; however, they can be viewed as benefiting the donor (e.g., praise, recognition, weight loss, increased self-awareness about health, increased self-awareness about mortality, optimized work–life balance and whole-person care, personal satisfaction for doing "good," and so on) Altruism, it seems, can have rewards.

It has been speculated that the intrinsic rewards of altruistic behavior promote such behavior toward strangers. Imagine if altruistic behavior boosted immunity, lengthened life span, created feelings of happiness, satisfaction and cooperation, and lowered stress. According to scientists, altruistic behavior *does* all of the above.[1] It would seem altruistic behavior is life's elixir! More correctly, it is the chemicals released during altruistic behavior that impact the life of the helper. For example, oxytocin is a hormone released by the pituitary (a small gland about the size of a pea that sits at the base of the brain). Oxytocin has been extensively studied and found to increase feelings of trust[2] and empathy[3] when administered in a nasal spray to research participants. Intranasal oxytocin has also been shown to reduce stress[4] and increase monetary donations under experimental conditions.[5] Similarly, progesterone (a hormone) is thought to be part of the neuroendocrine element of altruism, providing for the hormonal basis of social bonds (including oxytocin) that enable individuals to suppress self-interest when necessary in order to promote the well-being of others.[6] Progesterone and one of its metabolites (a small molecule produced when progesterone breaks down) are also involved in stress reduction, and thus progesterone could be part of a loop that both triggers and rewards altruistic behavior.

Another phenomena observed following altruistic behavior towards strangers is the "helper's high."[7] This is a two-phase event that starts out with a warm, rush release of endorphins (the body's natural pain relieving chemicals) that result in a physical "high" of good feeling and stress reduction, followed by a longer-lasting feeling of well-being, increased self-worth, peace, and calm.[8] As with progesterone, it seems that these chemical boosts could potentially create loops that both trigger and reward altruistic behavior. In other words, helping behavior could breed more helping behavior because of the mental and physical rewards to the helper (not to mention the genetic neural pathways in the brain that might facilitate the behavior).

Researchers have speculated that helpers see benefits to their own mental health because helping others gives the helper the opportunity to look outside their personal problems to see a new perspective on their own lives. In 2003, researchers at the University of Massachusetts Medical School reported the results of their study of altruism.[9] They asked more than 2,000 Presbyterians about their altruism practices as well as their mental and physical health. They found that those who engaged in helping activities had high mental health scores and that these scores were independent of the frequency of church attendance. "Significant predictors of giving help included endorsing more prayer activities, higher satisfaction with prayer life, engaging in positive religious coping, age, female gender, and being a church elder."[10] Participants got more out of giving than receiving; however, when they felt overburdened or asked to give beyond their resources, mental health scores dropped. This is why, as we discussed earlier, sometimes the timing or the activity might not be appropriate and the helper should not press forward, even if he or she feels a duty or destiny to help. Harm to helpers must always be part of the risk–benefit analysis.

THE "HIGH" OF ORGAN DONATION

As one of our donors told us, "Altruistic organ donation is the highest high than any human being could ever experience."[11] That being said, how can it be "topped"? Should donors try to top it with another high, or should they just bask in the joy of having helped another human? Living donation is not a conquest, nor is it a contest of physical strength or mental willpower; rather, it is an act of benevolence. Donors don't race against each other to see who will recover the fastest and who can donate the most organs. Nonetheless, for some donors, their first organ donation is sometimes not their last. Earlier, we discussed several donors who pursued evaluations for additional organ donations.

It is not uncommon for Good Samaritan donors to live in the limelight for a brief time after donating an organ. Television and newspaper reporters will sometimes camp out awaiting their first look at their city's "saint." This is because news of giving a vital organ to a stranger is exciting and rare as well as emotionally uplifting in times of crisis (e.g., war or economic despair). Media attention like this is not morally wrong; in fact, empathetic stories can motivate others to donate as either living or deceased donors. However, as discussed earlier, egoism and media interviews should not be the personal focus of those donating—altruism must be front and center. Any media attention that does happen is usually very short lived, often less than a week. It does not make anyone an "A-list" celebrity, nor should it. If there is any grandeur attached to organ donation, it is not about the donors but about their *gift*.

Some Good Samaritan donors have embraced the media as a tool to promote organ donation. Lori Palatnik, the wife of a rabbi, originally planned to give a kidney to a friend but found out she was too small to size match to him (he was a lot larger and would need a bigger kidney). Lori was not deterred. She had been involved in organizing a bone marrow drive before and knew that matches, in general, can take some effort. She responded to a general plea for living donors, was tested and matched, and donated to a woman (her "kidney sister") in New York in 2007. She subsequently posted a four-part YouTube video on the Internet that tells her story and promotes the cause.[12] In New York, Good Samaritan kidney donor Chaya Lipschutz created a YouTube channel devoted to organ donation.[13] There she has uploaded videos chronicling donations and transplants from around the world. In our clinical experience, some donor candidates seek to have their donor surgeries filmed in the operating room. The purpose for this can vary. Some donors want a video for personal reflection: to watch and commemorate their experience. Others want to use the video as part of a larger film production effort, such as a documentary about organ donation. Requests for surgical filming are handled on a case-by-case basis by transplant hospitals. Donor teams must ensure that there is no egocentric motive for filming (e.g., donor seeks to become a "star" and make money from presupposed film profits).

At least two of our Good Samaritan donors have had their cases published in medical journals. This is not a form of "stardom" for the donor; rather, this transmission of clinical information is standard educational practice for physicians. In both of these cases, they were a "first" for their country: the first Good Samaritan liver donation in Belgium[14] and the first Good Samaritan kidney donation in Canada.[15] Pioneering medical efforts are commonly reported at national and international conferences as well as in medical journals. Articles such as these serve many purposes, including "breaking the ice" so that other physicians can feel comfortable following a leader, educating physicians and surgeons about techniques and risks, and providing hospitals and related organizations with guidance to assist with the establishment or revision of policy. Medical journal case reports require the consent of the donor for publication, and no compensation is received by either the donor or the author who writes the article.

Most of the Good Samaritan donors we interviewed told us that their lives had not changed much after their donation. They returned to their jobs, hobbies, and family roles. A rare few had medical side effects. Two of twenty-two donors lost weight after their donation and kept it off, maintaining a healthy weight profile for their stature. Six of twenty-two donors reported being more aware of their health, taking care of themselves better, and having better health than before donation. Good Samaritan donors generally already have the inclination to "eat right," exercise, and avoid excessive stress and destructive behaviors (e.g., use of tobacco, excessive alcohol, or recreational drugs) before their donation, and they carry on these inclinations afterward.

Life after surgery can be unnerving and disappointing for some Good Samaritan donors. This is because some donors feel that they were minimally valued in terms of laying their life on the line for others. They sometimes also feel that their donations were undervalued by the transplant team or the organ recipients. These reactions have been seen in both Good Samaritan donors as well as those donating to relatives. In 2006, researchers from Harvard Medical School reported a study of fifteen living lung donors.[16] These donors participated in open-ended interviews with a psychiatrist to give follow up on their donation experience. Quoting the researchers, "As a group, the subjective impression imparted by the donors . . . was that they wished for greater acknowledgment of their role in the transplant process."[17] Most of the donors felt that the value of their donation was not embraced by either the organ recipient or the team. When two donor–recipient pairs were interviewed together as part of a press conference, the donors felt that the recipients overshadowed them. Donors also were upset when their recipients did not seek them out or acknowledge the special relationship that inherently exists between the two. The two donors who were interviewed for newspaper articles were the only donors who reported feeling appreciated for their personal sacrifice. In another research study, thirty-nine individuals who had donated kidneys to friends or family members in Sweden were interviewed.[18] Of these, 28 percent reported feeling "abandoned, exploited, and ignored by the staff."[19] One donor commented feeling pressured to leave the hospital (as though awaiting eviction) so that another patient could use the bed. Another indicated the care abruptly changed *after* donation—staff were less responsive to needs.

In our group of twenty-two Good Samaritan donors, the majority felt that they were well taken care of and appreciated by the donor team, with one indicating that his hospital treated him like a "rock star."[20] But, similar to the Swedish study discussed above, 27 percent of our donors reported dissatisfaction with elements of their immediate postdonation life. One donor commented that while he was in the custody of the hospital, he was treated with great care and respect and that any concerns were promptly addressed. However, on discharge, he was at home getting the "silent treatment" from the donor team when he phoned them with questions. Quoting him, he felt as if the attitude of the hospital was, "Well we got your kidney; we don't need you anymore."[21] Another individual who donated a kidney (at a different hospital) had a very similar experience as just described.[22] A liver donor commented that he felt he was discharged from the hospital too soon.[23] He didn't feel ready to leave. And when he did leave, he felt "dropped."[24] This individual has concerns that donors not be forgotten ("Don't just take their organ!").[25] A kidney donor in our group was perplexed and irritated by the fact that her surgeon never came by to check on her or phone her while she was recovering in the hospital. Other team members monitored her recovery progress, but she never saw her own surgeon after the nephrectomy. When she finally met up with him during an outpatient postoperative checkup, the surgeon did not recognize her and had a "cavalier" attitude, inquiring of her, "Have we met?"[26] One donor's sleep was so disrupted by his hospital roommate that he crawled on his hands and knees (after liver donation) from his room to a family waiting room down the hall in the middle of the night so that he could get some peaceful rest.

Clearly, these negative situations are disturbing. To help make living donors feel valued, some hospitals give them "VIP treatment," such as large, private rooms with views, but this can be superficial "thanks." Donor teams need to adopt a global attitude of caring *and* appreciation, as both promote donor welfare. Organ donors don't want a hospital floor named after them—that is not the recognition they are seeking. They do seek—and it is appropriate to give them—respect for their beneficent act, quality medical follow-up care, and continued general monitoring of their outcome. As one donor stated, there is a lack of "moral follow up"—individuals should be checked on to see how they are coping physically and psychosocially after their living donation.[27] Showing donors that they are valued does not detract from the altruistic nature of the donation. Similarly, a desire to be valued by the team (or society in general) does not equate to a pathological desire for recognition. Individuals should not be treated like their organs are commodities, and they should not have to beg for needed medical attention after donation.

MORE GOOD WORKS

It seems that the altruistic trends that preceded organ donation continue even afterward. Several of those we interviewed remain blood donors and potential marrow donors (they are registered and awaiting a match to a needy patient). Jeff, a Good Samaritan kidney donor in Ohio, is typical of many of the donors we interviewed.[28] Prior to organ donation, this man (blind since childhood) had been active for many years in the disability rights arena, working with technology and legislation to facilitate widespread use of Remote Infrared Audible Signage for the visually impaired. (The technology consists of a transmitter that continuously emits an infrared beam that can be picked up with a small handheld receiver. Individuals scan the environment with the receiver and intercept the infrared beam, which contains a voice message that is heard through the receiver's speaker. The voice informs the listener what is in the environment and also gives directions.) After donation, Jeff was plagued by months of nausea. Having no regrets about his decision to donate, Jeff is working to form a donor mentoring group that will consist of former living donors (all organ types) that network together to discuss their needs and obtain emotional support, educational information, and resource referrals. Jeff wants no donor to feel alone after the donation, especially if the donor has a complication. Additionally, Jeff has written a song about organ donation and plans to write a book about his experience.

Nicole was so thrilled with her Good Samaritan kidney donation experience that she formed the Christian Kidney Foundation.[29] She and her husband travel to churches and other events to educate people about organ donation. Arlene, also a kidney donor, continues to ride her motorcycle in charity events that benefit various disease foundations and animal shelters.[30] Another kidney donor, Matthew, volunteers his time to the "No One Dies Alone Program."[31] With this national program, each patient has someone to spend their last days and hours with so that they have the dignity of not being alone at the time they pass away. Dave, a lung lobe donor, participated in a charity event climbing the stairs of the tallest office building in San Diego (thirty-two floors) in an effort to raise money for the Cystic Fibrosis Foundation.[32] Chad, a kidney donor in Utah, donated an old car to the National Kidney Foundation.[33] Scott, a kidney donor, participated in the 2011 Polar Plunge and raised nearly $500 for the Wisconsin Special Olympics when he jumped into the frigid Mississippi River.[34] Beneficent acts continue throughout their lives.

But how do our twenty-two Good Samaritan donors feel about advocating for *others* to be living organ donors? Do they bang drums and wave flags to promote the practice? We asked them about this concept and got a mixed response. Fourteen donors indicated that they spoke about donation with others and promoted it, but eight indicated otherwise. For this latter group, it is not that they are unhappy with their donation experience; rather, they feel that living donation is a personal matter and not suited for everyone, so they don't actively promote the concept. Others in this group of eight don't talk about living donation unless someone brings up the topic or asks about their experience—they prefer to keep the matter private. None of our twenty-two donors indicated that they have changed their mind about the beneficence of organ donation.

In Matthew's words, "I didn't donate the kidney for praise."[35] He feels that living donation is an "extraordinary thing" and because of that, it is not for everyone. He chooses not to talk about his donation unless someone else mentions it or seriously asks him about his opinion. In those situations, he feels that the inquiry is an attempt by someone to seek out information because they have the bona fide intent to do a good deed; thus, he has no hesitation to tell them that they need only one of their two kidneys. Ken, a Good Samaritan liver donor, takes a broader approach, telling everyone he can about organ donation. He gives talks at community groups and has a personal philosophy about living donation: "You don't know what you're missing!"[36]

For those living donors who are athletically inclined, a unique opportunity is now available in the United States. Beginning in 2010, the U.S. Transplant Games included living donor participants (in addition to organ transplant patients).[37] To qualify, individuals who have given any vital organ or bone marrow and who are healthy and at least nine months postdonation may participate. During the nearly weeklong competition, living donors contend against each other in the following events: men's and women's 5K race, 100-meter dash, ball throw, and long jump. Judy Payne, a fifty-nine-year-old Good Samaritan donor from Virginia, won the women's 5K race. She has a long history of marathon running and continues racking up the miles even after her kidney donation to a stranger. Another sporting event for living donors is the "MiniMarathon" (5K race) sponsored by the World Transplant Games.[38] In 2011, the race was held in Göteborg, Sweden, and in 2013, the race will be held in Durban, South Africa. The purpose of these athletic events is to bring donors together in social fellowship as well as to show the world their physical prowess. The latter is an excellent witness about the general safety of living donation.

· 30 ·

Elevation

$\mathscr{T}$hroughout this book, we've tried to present a balanced picture of living donation. There are risks and there are benefits. Donor candidates should never downplay or underestimate the risks and should take them seriously, reflecting on them in the context of their personal situation, including their medical history, emotional stamina, personal relationships, and financial health. On balance, we conclude that living donation has a risk–benefit profile that renders it an ethically appropriate technology, but it is not appropriate for everyone. For some, the altruistic act that is most fitting for them is blood, platelet, or marrow donation, whereas for others, it might be volunteer work with the elderly, infirmed, or incarcerated. All these prosocial behaviors make the world a better place.

As we discussed earlier, the performance of prosocial acts toward strangers can result in a phenomena termed the "helper's high."[1] Initially, the helper feels a warm, rush release of endorphins that result in a physical "high" of good feeling and stress reduction. This is followed by a longer-lasting feeling of well-being, increased self-worth, peace, and calm. Researchers suspect that these chemical boosts could potentially create circuits that both trigger and reward altruistic behavior, meaning that helping behavior could propagate more helping behavior because of the rewards to the helper.

"Elevation" is another unique but related phenomena. With elevation, the *observation* of another person performing in a "virtuous, pure, or super-human way"[2] causes profound emotional and physical reactions in the observer. Emotional reactions[3] include a desire to help others, a desire to become a bet-ter person, feeling inspired and uplifted, setting higher goals for oneself, feeling more optimistic about the view of humanity, having a desire to be with people and love them, and a desire to "emulate the exemplar."[4] The most common physical symptoms are a warm, pleasant, tingling feeling in the chest.[5] To be clear, elevation is not the same as joy, happiness, or admiration. It is much more complex than that. In fact, the key feature of elevation is that observers turn their attention *away from themselves* and outward toward others. This is why elevation is linked to altruism. Admiration, on the other hand, is linked not to the viewing of virtuous acts (moral excellence) but rather to general acts of accomplishment (nonmoral excellence) such as athletic feats (e.g., a large quantity of home run hits in baseball or world-record sprinting or swimming). Admiration may generate positive emotional feelings for the observer, but it does not generally result in the observer turning outward and performing acts of prosocial behavior toward others.[6] This is unique to elevation.

Thomas Jefferson was the first person to formally discuss the concept of elevation. In 1771 when he was working as an inventor, architect, and attorney (thirty years before his role as U.S. president), he wrote a letter to his brother-in-law stating, "When any . . . act of charity or of gratitude, for instance, is presented either to our sight or imagination, we are deeply impressed with its beauty and feel a strong desire in ourselves of doing charitable and grateful acts also."[7] He then wondered, in a rhetorical tone, whether circulated accounts of virtuous action "do not dilate [the reader's] breast, and elevate his sentiments as much as any similar incident which real history can furnish?"[8] It seems that dilation of the breast would be consistent with the warm, pleasant feeling in the chest we spoke of earlier.

More than 200 years went by before psychologists began studying the concept of elevation. While the field of elevation research is relatively new (less than fifteen years old), there have been some interesting findings. For example, when people were divided into groups and shown either a documentary about Mother Theresa, comedy videos, or emotionally neutral documentaries, those who watched the Mother Theresa documentary were more likely to experience elevation and were more likely to volunteer at a humanitarian charity organization afterward.[9] In another study,[10] students from four U.S. universities spent time with orphans in Nicaragua on a weeklong service trip. Elevation resulted in the tendency for volunteerism on topics related to the trip after the return home.

According to the world's expert on elevation, psychologist Jonathan Haidt, the most common circumstances that elicit elevation are the observation of someone giving help to the poor or sick or those stranded in difficult situations.[11] While all our Good Samaritan donor interviews were conducted after the fact, and we were not present to test for elevation on the day they decided to become donors, we can look at the historical information they provided us with about their donation experiences. In doing so, we found that 36 percent of our Good Samaritan donors gave their gift as a result of observing living organ donation by another person. Specifically, four donors watched television stories about Good Samaritan donation, three donors read books or newspaper articles about Good Samaritan or living donation, and one donor had a relative participate as a living donor. These results correlate with the work of psychology researcher Keith Cox, who has concluded that elevation can predict domain-specific volunteerism.[12] Specifically, when people are elevated by observing a particular activity, they tend to respond by volunteering in a domain (e.g., illness, geriatrics, pediatrics, or the incarcerated) related to that activity rather than something unrelated to what was observed. This is not to say that thousands more people watched the same television programs and read the same books and newspaper articles that our donors did, experienced elevation, and did *other* acts of prosocial behavior. This could very well be the case. As we continue to stress, organ donation is not for everybody, and there are many ways to contribute to society.

Another interesting feature of elevation is the fact that it has the potential to cause a domino effect, a cascade of prosocial behaviors. In this way, elevation can be contagious. (Thomas Jefferson already knew that.)[13] The more acts of prosocial behavior in the world, the more beneficence gets spread around. This results in a decrease in suffering. We hope that the donor profiles we have shared spark elevation in our readers. And we hope that our exploration of altruism in these donors helps calm some of the fears of transplant professionals. As we have shown, good screening can select for appropriate donors. Our goal is to see the patient waiting list shrink as more people sign up to be deceased organ donors on their death[14] and more people participate as living donors to friends, family, and even strangers.

If all humans belong to one family
are there really any strangers?
A Good Samaritan will tell you,
What's mine is yours.

Appendix: Living Donor Resources

WEBSITES

American Liver Foundation	http://www.liverfoundation.org
American Red Cross	http://www.redcross.org
American Society of Transplantation	http://www.healthy-donor.com
Donate Life America	http://www.donatelife.net
Euro Living Donor	http://www.eulivingdonor.eu
Halachic Organ Donor Society	http://www.hods.org
International Assoc. of Living Organ Donors	http://www.livingdonorsonline.org
Kidney Foundation of Canada	http://www.kidney.ca
Living Donor 101	http://www.livingdonor101.com
Living Donor Advocate Program	http://www.lodap.com
Living Organ Donation in Europe	http://www.eulod.eu
National Kidney Foundation	http://www.kidney.org
National Kidney Registry	http://www.kidneyregistry.org
National Living Donor Assistance Center	http://www.livingdonorassistance.org
Second Wind Lung Transplant Association	http://www.2ndwind.org
Transplant Buddies	http://www.transplantbuddies.org
Transplant Ethics	http://www.transplantethics.com
United Network for Organ Sharing	http://www.transplantliving.org

READING MATERIAL

To access the medical journal articles we have referenced in the book, visit your local hospital's patient library and speak to the librarian for assistance. You can also visit your nearest university library. The local public library generally does not have medical journal holdings, but the librarian can help you order articles. Some articles are available free via PubMed Central (http://www.ncbi.nlm.nih.gov/pmc) or the publisher. Another method is contacting the corresponding author and asking for a reprint. Often, the mailing address and the email address of the author are noted near the article's abstract.

Notes

INTRODUCTION

1. United Network for Organ Sharing, "Data," accessed December 23, 2010, http://www.unos.org.

2. Ibid.

3. Ibid.

4. Ibid.

5. Personal communication between Arlene Arthur (donor) and Rena Down (recipient), San Francisco, June 5, 2005.

6. Sam Whiting, "Transplant Ethicist Guards Organ Donors' Rights," *San Francisco Chronicle*, March 23, 2009, accessed December 23, 2010, http://www.cpmc.org/advanced/kidney/news/Bramstedt.pdf.

7. Personal communication, San Francisco, June 12, 2009.

8. Personal communication, Lima, Peru, May 15, 2005.

9. Ibid.

10. http://www.Craigslist.com.

11. Personal communication, Arthur and Down, June 5, 2005.

12. Ibid.

13. Ibid.

CHAPTER 1: ETHICS, VALUES, MOTIVATIONS

1. Public Law 98-507, Title III, Section 301a. "Prohibition of Organ Purchases."

2. Oxford Dictionaries, s.v. "*altruism*," accessed October 18, 2010, http://oxford dictionairies.com.

3. Luke 10:25–37.

4. Samuel P. Oliner and Pearl M. Oliner, *The Altruistic Personality: Rescuers of Jews in Nazi Europe* (New York: Free Press, 1988), 3.

5. Lawrence Kohlberg, "Moral Stages and Moralization: The Cognitive-Developmental Approach," in *Moral Development and Behavior: Theory, Research, and Social Issues*, ed. Tom Lickona (New York: Holt, Rinehart & Winston, 1976), 31–53.

6. Ervin Staub, "Helping a Distressed Person: Social, Personality, and Stimulus Determinants," in *Advances in Experimental Social Psychology*, ed. Leonard Berkowitz (New York: Academic Press, 1974), vol. 7, 293–341.

7. Shaun Nichols, "Mindreading and the Cognitive Architecture Underlying Altruistic Motivation," *Mind & Language* 16 (2001): 425–55.

8. Ken Schuler, telephone interview with Katrina Bramstedt, January 31, 2010.

9. C. Daniel Batson and Laura L. Shaw, "Evidence for Altruism: Toward a Pluralism of Prosocial Motives," *Psychological Inquiry* 2, no. 2 (1991): 107–22.

10. Ibid., 108.

11. *Organ Donation*, SB 1395, State of California (September 2, 2010).

12. H. Harrison Sadler et al., "The Living, Genetically Unrelated, Kidney Donor," *Seminars in Psychiatry* 3 (1971): 86–101.

13. Ibid., 96.

14. Ibid.

15. Ibid., 89.

16. Ibid., 91.

17. Ibid., 93.

18. Ibid.

19. Ibid., 99.

20. Ibid., 89–91.

21. Ibid., 97.

22. Antonio a J. Z. Henderson et al., "The Living Anonymous Kidney Donor: Lunatic or Saint?" *American Journal of Transplantation* 3, no. 2 (2003): 203–13.

23. Paul S. Mueller, Ellen J. Case, and C. Christopher Hook, "Responding to Offers of Altruistic Living Unrelated Kidney Donation by Group Associations: An Ethical Analysis," *Transplantation Reviews* 22, no. 3 (2008): 200–205; David J. Dixon and Susan E. Abbey, "Religious Altruism and the Living Organ Donor," *Progress in Transplantation* 13, no. 3 (2003): 169–75; Reginald Y. Gohh et al., "Controversies in Organ Donation: The Altruistic Living Donor," *Nephrology, Dialysis, Transplantation* 16, no. 3 (2001): 619–21.

24. Henderson et al., 206; M. D. Jendrisak et al., "Altruistic Living Donors: Evaluation for Nondirected Kidney or Liver Donation," *American Journal of Transplantation* 6, no. 1 (2006): 115–20; E. K. Massey et al., "Encouraging Psychological Outcomes after Altruistic Donation to a Stranger," *American Journal of Transplantation* 10, no. 6 (2010): 1445–52.

25. Massey et al., "Encouraging Psychological Outcomes,"1447.

26. Judy Esmond and Patrick Dunlop, "Developing the Volunteer Motivation Inventory to Assess the Underlying Motivational Drives of Volunteers in Western Australia," 2004, pp. 71–72, accessed October 18, 2010, http://mtd4u.com/resources/MotivationFinalReport.pdf.

27. Luke 10:25–29.

28. John Wilson and Marc Musick, *Volunteers: A Social Profile* (Bloomington: Indiana University Press, 2008), 42–50.

29. Mark Davis, "Measuring Individual Differences in Empathy: Evidence for a Multidimensional Approach," *Journal of Personality and Social Psychology* 44, no. 1 (1983): 113–24.

30. Wilson and Musick, *Volunteers*, 44.

31. Ibid., 46.

32. Ibid., 45.

33. "KidneyMitzvah.com," Chaya Lipschutz, accessed October 18, 2010, http://kidneymitzvah.com.

34. Wilson and Musick, *Volunteers*, 77.

35. Jerry Z. Park and Christian Smith, "'To Whom Much Has Been Given . . . ': Religious Capital and Community Voluntarism among Churchgoing Protestants," *Journal for the Scientific Study of Religion* 39, no. 3 (2000): 272–86.

CHAPTER 2: FRED

1. Northeast Family Federal Credit Union, "Credit Union Man," accessed December 14, 2010, http://creditunionman.com.

2. "Rotary International," accessed December 14, 2010, http://www.rotary.org.

3. Rotary International, "Polio," accessed December 14, 2010, http://www.rotary.org/en/ServiceAndFellowship/Polio/Pages/ridefault.aspx.

4. Rotaplast International, "Rotaplast: Saving Smiles, Changing Lives," accessed December 14, 2010, http://www.rotaplast.org.

5. "LifePlant International," accessed December 14, 2010, http://www.rotaplant.com.

6. Fred Brown, telephone interview with Katrina Bramstedt, January 30, 2010.

7. Ibid.

8. Eyewitness News 3, "Man Donates Kidney to Complete Stranger," December 4, 2009, accessed January 29, 2010, http://www.wfsb.com/health/21866354/detail.html.

9. "Local Man Gives a Patient the Gift of Life," *RxTra*, 65, no. 52, December 2009, accessed December 15, 2010, http://www.harthosp.org/Portals/1/Images/6/rxtra/Dec-2009.pdf.

10. Brown, interview with Bramstedt, January 30, 2010.

CHAPTER 3: JOSIE

1. U.S. Department of Health and Human Services Office of Minority Health, "Organ Donation and Asian Americans," August 3, 2010, accessed December 13, 2010, http://minorityhealth.hhs.gov/templates/content.aspx?lvl=3&lvlID=12&ID=7991.

2. Josie Soriano, telephone interview with Rena Down, August 15, 2009.

3. "National Kidney Registry," accessed December 13, 2010, http://www.kidney registry.org.

4. Stanford Hospital and Clinics, "A Positive Chain Reaction: The Sorianos One Year Later," accessed December 13, 2010, http://stanfordhospital.org/newsEvents/ newsReleases/2009/sorianosoneyearlater.html.

5. Soriano, interview with Down, August 15, 2009.

6. Ibid.

CHAPTER 4: MATT

1. Matt Auchter, interview by Rena Down, Marriott Hotel, Philadelphia, October 5, 2009.

2. Ibid.

3. Ibid.

4. Ibid.

5. Ibid.

6. Ibid.

7. Ibid.

8. Matthew Auchter, telephone interview with Rena Down, August 10, 2009.

9. Ibid.

10. Ibid.

11. Auchter, interview by Down, October 5, 2009.

12. Auchter, interview with Down, August 10, 2009.

13. Ibid.

14. Ibid.

15. Ibid.

16. Ibid.

CHAPTER 5: CONSTRUCTS OF DESTINY

1. David J. Dixon and Susan E. Abbey, "Religious Altruism and the Living Organ Donor," *Progress in Transplantation* 13, no. 3 (2003): 169–75.

2. Ibid., 171–72.

3. Paul S. Mueller, Ellen J. Case, and C. Christopher Hook, "Responding to Offers of Altruistic Living Unrelated Kidney Donation by Group Associations: An Ethical Analysis," *Transplantation Reviews* 22, no. 3 (2008): 200–205.

4. "Kidneys," Jesus Christians, accessed October 28, 2008, http://www.jesus teachings.com/kidneys.

5. Ibid.

6. Reginald Y. Gohh et al., "Controversies in Organ Donation: The Altruistic Living Donor," *Nephrology, Dialysis, Transplantation* 16, no. 3 (2001): 619–21.

7. Ibid., 621.

8. Dave Manglos, telephone interview with Katrina Bramstedt, February 1, 2010.

9. Ibid.

10. Cheryl Brennan, telephone interview with Katrina Bramstedt, January 23, 2010.

11. Max Zapata, telephone interview with Katrina Bramstedt, February 6, 2010.

12. Ibid.

13. Jeff Moyer, telephone interview with Katrina Bramstedt, July 28, 2010.

14. Ibid.

15. Ibid.

16. Jack Marschall, telephone interview with Rena Down, August 22, 2009.

17. Ibid.

18. Ibid.

19. Olav Rueppell, M. K. Hayworth, and N. P. Ross, "Altruistic Self-Removal of Health-Compromised Honey Bee Workers from Their Hive," *Journal of Evolutionary Biology* 23, no. 7 (2010): 1538–46.

20. C. Bordereau et al., "Suicidal Defensive Behaviour by Frontal Gland Dehiscence in *Globitermes sulphureus* Haviland Soldiers (Isoptera)," *Insectes Sociaux* 44, no. 3 (1997): 289–96.

21. Richard C. Connor and Kenneth S. Norris, "Are Dolphins Reciprocal Altruists?," *American Naturalist* 199, no. 3 (1982): 358–74.

22. Martin Reuter et al., "Investigating the Genetic Basis of Altruism: The Role of the COMT Val158Met Polymorphism," *Social Cognitive and Affective Neuroscience*, October 28, 2010 [Epub ahead of print].

23. Vani A. Mathur et al., "Neural Basis of Extraordinary Empathy and Altruistic Motivation," *NeuroImage* 51, no. 4 (2010): 1468–75.

24. Ariel Knafo and Robert Plomin, "Parental Discipline and Affection and Children's Prosocial Behavior: Genetic and Environmental Links," *Journal of Personality and Social Psychology* 90, no. 1 (2006): 147–64; Samuel P. Oliner and Pearl M. Oliner, *The Altruistic Personality: Rescuers of Jews in Nazi Europe* (New York: Free Press, 1988), 3.

25. J. Philippe Rushton, "Is Altruism Innate?" *Psychological Inquiry* 2 (1991): 141–43.

26. Felix Warneken and Michael Tomasello, "The Roots of Human Altruism," *British Journal of Psychology* 100, pt. 3 (2009): 455–71.

27. Ibid.

28. Judy Esmond and Patrick Dunlop, "Developing the Volunteer Motivation Inventory to Assess the Underlying Motivational Drives of Volunteers in Western Australia," 2004, pp. 71–72, accessed October 18, 2010, http://mtd4u.com/resources/MotivationFinalReport.pdf.

29. 42 CFR 482.98(d) (2009).

CHAPTER 6: DAVE

1. Dave Manglos, telephone interview with Katrina Bramstedt, February 1, 2010.

2. Keith Schneider, "Plane Crash in Georgia Kills 23, Including Former Senator Tower," *New York Times*, April 6, 1991, accessed December 9, 2010, http://www

.nytimes.com/1991/04/06/us/plane-crash-in-georgia-kills-23-including-former
-senator-tower.html.

3. "Senator John Goodwin Tower Dies in Plane Crash," accessed December 8, 2010, http://avstop.com/news/senatortower.html.

4. Mary Brown, "I'll Go Where You Want Me to Go," 1899.

5. Ibid., note 1.

6. Roland Merullo, "Every Breath He Takes," *Reader's Digest*, December 2003, accessed December 8, 2010, http://www.rd.com/content/printContent.do?conte ntId=28562&KeepThis=true&TB_iframe=true&height=500&width=790&modal =true.

CHAPTER 7: CHERYL

1. Cheryl Brennan, telephone interview with Katrina Bramstedt, January 23, 2010.

2. Ibid.

3. Ibid.

4. Ibid.

5. Ibid.

6. Ibid.

7. Ibid.

CHAPTER 8: MAX

1. Max Zapata, telephone interview with Katrina Bramstedt, February 6, 2010.

2. Ibid.

3. In answer to a question asked by the editors of *Youth*, a journal of Young Israel of Williamsburg, New York; quoted in the *New York Times*, June 20, 1932; *Einstein Archive* 60–492, 1932.

4. Personal email communication from Max Zapata, December 21, 2010.

5. U.S. Department of Health and Human Services Office of Minority Health, "Organ Donation and Hispanic Americans," August 3, 2010, accessed December 3, 2010, http://minorityhealth.hhs.gov/templates/content .aspx?lvl=3&lvlID=12&ID=7989.

6. Ibid.

7. Ibid.

8. Zapata, interview with Bramstedt, February 6, 2010.

9. Ibid.

10. "Dance for Donors," accessed December 4, 2010, http://www.dancefordo nors.org.

11. Katie Couric, "Kidney Chains Link Total Strangers Saving Lives," November 10, 2010, accessed December 3, 2010, http://www.cbsnews.com/stories/2010/11/10/ eveningnews/main7042117.shtml.

CHAPTER 9: JEFF

1. Jeff Moyer, telephone interview with Katrina Bramstedt, July 28, 2010.

2. Jeff Moyer, "Music from the Heart: Jeff Moyer," accessed December 10, 2010, http://www.jeffmoyer.com.

3. Liz Hull, "Mother, 81, Becomes Oldest Living Kidney Donor with a Gift of Life to Her Son," *Mail Online*, April 30, 2008, accessed December 1, 2010, http:// www.dailymail.co.uk/news/article-563037/Mother-81-oldest-living-kidney-donor -gift-life-son.html#ixzz16szTkPxm.

4. Ibid., note 1.

5. Ibid.

6. Ibid.

7. Jeff Moyer, "Selected" (Cleveland, OH: Music From the Heart, 2010).

8. Ibid., note 1.

9. Jeff Moyer, "Giving a Kidney, Gaining a Lifelong Friend," *National Public Radio*, September13, 2010, accessed December 10, 2010, http://www.npr.org/tem-plates/story/story.php?storyId=129731335.

10. Moyer, interview with Bramstedt, July 28, 2010.

11. Ibid.

12. Moyer, "Music from the Heart."

CHAPTER 10: JACK

1. Paired Donation Network, "PDN, Paired Donation Network," accessed December 6, 2010, http://www.paireddonationnetwork.org/Default.aspx.

2. Eric Mull, "Jack and Lauren Marschall," January 2008, accessed December 6, 2010, http://www.clevelandmagazine.com/ME2/dirmod.asp?sid=E73ABD6180B44 874871A91F6BA5C249C&nm=Arts+%26+Entertainemnt&type=Publishing&mod= Publications%3A%3AArticle&mid=1578600D80804596A222593669321019&tier=4 &id=1EDC917B0F6A498380E494B468A10115.

3. Jack Marschall, telephone interview with Rena Down, August 22, 2009.

4. Ibid.

5. Ibid.

6. Ibid.

7. Ibid.

8. Ibid.

9. Library of Congress, "The September 11, 2001, Web Archive," accessed December 6, 2010, http://lcweb2.loc.gov/diglib/lcwa/html/sept11/sept11-overview.html.

10. Marschall, interview with Down, August 22, 2009.

CHAPTER 11: TRENDS AMONG GOOD SAMARITANS

1. Nicole Lanstrum, telephone interview with Rena Down, August 10, 2009.

2. David Rosenhan, "The Natural Socialization of Altruistic Autonomy," in *Altruism and Helping Behavior*, ed. Jacqueline Macaulay and Leonard Berkowitz (New York: Academic Press, 1970).

3. E. K. Massey et al., "Encouraging Psychological Outcomes after Altruistic Donation to a Stranger," *American Journal of Transplantation* 10, no. 6 (2010): 1447; Antonioa J. Z. Henderson et al., "The Living Anonymous Kidney Donor: Lunatic or Saint?," *American Journal of Transplantation* 3, no. 2 (2003): 207.

4. T. W. Reichman et al., "Anonymous Living Liver Donation: Donor Profiles and Outcomes," *American Journal of Transplantation* 10, no. 9 (2010): 2101.

5. Karen Ormiston, telephone interview with Rena Down, August 26, 2009.

6. Nicole Lanstrum, telephone interview with Rena Down, August 10, 2009.

7. Fred Brown, telephone interview with Katrina Bramstedt, January 30, 2010.

8. Maureen Vavro, telephone interview with Rena Down, October 17, 2009.

9. Jack Marschall, telephone interview with Rena Down, August 22, 2009.

10. Deborah Craigo, telephone interview with Rena Down, October 31, 2009.

11. Max Zapata, telephone interview with Katrina Bramstedt, February 6, 2010.

12. Judy Esmond and Patrick Dunlop, "Developing the Volunteer Motivation Inventory to Assess the Underlying Motivational Drives of Volunteers in Western Australia," 2004, p. 74, accessed October 18, 2010, http://mtd4u.com/resources/MotivationFinalReport.pdf.

13. Ibid., 71–72.

14. U.S. Department of Health and Human Services Organ Procurement and Transplant Network Organ Distribution Policy 3.5.11.6, "Donation Status," United Network for Organ Sharing, November 9, 2010, accessed October 13, 2010, http://optn.transplant.hrsa.gov/policiesAndBylaws/policies.asp.

15. Garrett Gall, telephone interview with Rena Down, October 4, 2009.

16. Cynthia Marshall, interviewed by Rena Down, August 14, 2009.

17. John Wilson and Marc Musick, *Volunteers: A Social Profile* (Bloomington: Indiana University Press, 2008), 98–101.

18. Dave Manglos, telephone interview with Katrina Bramstedt, February 1, 2010.

19. Cheryl Brennan, telephone interview with Katrina Bramstedt, January 23, 2010.

20. Nicole Lanstrum, interviewed by Rena Down.

21. The identity of this donor is anonymized in this instance so as to not alarm the recipient. This interview was conducted telephonically by Rena Down on August 15, 2009.

22. Max Zapata, telephone interview with Katrina Bramstedt, February 6, 2010.

23. Janet Lavelle, "San Diego Couple Final Link in Kidney Transplant Chain," *San Diego Union-Tribune*, August 28, 2010, accessed October 28, 2010, http://www.signon sandiego.com/news/2010/aug/27/san-diego-couple-participates-nations-largest-kidn.

24. Tim Bayne and Neil Levy, "Amputees by Choice: Body Integrity Identity Disorder and the Ethics of Amputation," *Journal of Applied Philosophy* 22, no. 1 (2005): 75–86.

25. Ian Parker, "The Gift: Zell Kravinsky Gave Away Millions: But Somehow It Wasn't Enough," *New Yorker*, August 2, 2004, 54–63.

CHAPTER 12: DEBORAH

1. Deborah Craigo, telephone interview with Rena Down, October 31, 2009.

2. Ibid.

3. Dan Patrone, "Disfigured Anatomies and Imperfect Analogies: Body Integrity Identity Disorder and the Supposed Right to Self-Demanded Amputation of Healthy Body Parts," *Journal of Medical Ethics* 35, no. 9 (2009): 541–45.

4. Craigo, interview with Down, October 31, 2009.

5. Ibid.

6. Ibid.

7. Ibid.

8. Ibid.

9. Ibid.

CHAPTER 13: MISSY

1. Missy Simpson, telephone interview with Katrina Bramstedt, January 21, 2010.

2. Marc Ian Barasch, *Field Notes on a Compassionate Life: A Search for the Soul of Kindness* (New York: Rodale, 2005), 147–202.

3. Simpson, interview with Bramstedt, January 21, 2010.

4. Martha Simpson, "If You Can't Donate" (unpublished manuscript), November 13, 2006.

5. Ibid.

6. Simpson, interview with Bramstedt, January 21, 2010.

7. Ibid.

CHAPTER 14: SAINTS OR NORMAL FOLK?

1. Yonit Tanenbaum, "Rabbi's Kidney Donation Inspires Community," August 20, 2009, accessed November 8, 2010, http://www.chabad.org/news/article_cdo/aid/968210/jewish/Rabbi-Gives-Gift-of-Life.htm.

2. Jotham Sederstrom, "Ground Zero Worker in Rare Kidney Swap Set to Exit Hospital," September 2, 2007, accessed November 8, 2010, http://www.nydailynews.com/news/2007/09/02/2007-09-02_ground_zero_worker_in_rare_kidney_swap_s.html.

3. Ibid.; John Feal, "The FealGoodFoundation," accessed November 8, 2010, http://www.fealgoodfoundation.com.

4. In a paired donation transplant, there are two donor–recipient pairs, which, as individual sets, are immunologically incompatible. Neither donor can give to his or her originally planned recipient, so the two pairs are shuffled, creating two immunologically compatible ("matching") pairs.

5. Joe Rosner, *Street Smarts & Self-Defense for Children: A Parent's Guide* (Seattle: CreateSpace, 2009).

6. "Best Defense USA," accessed November 11, 2010, http://bestdefenseillinois.com/home.

7. Carolyn Starks, "A Resident's Gift Changes Life of Stranger," *Chicago Tribune*, January 30, 2009, accessed November 11, 2010, http://articles.chicagotribune.com/2009-01-30/news/0901290786_1_national-kidney-foundation-donated-multiple-sclerosis.

8. "Barista Donates Kidney to Save Customer's Life," March 27, 2008, accessed November 16, 2010, http://articles.cnn.com/2008-03-27/living/heroes.andersen_1_kidney-transplant-kidney-disease-barista?_s=PM:LIVING.

9. "Church Janitor Donates Kidney to Stranger," December 24, 2008, accessed November 17, 2010, http://www.youtube.com/watch?v=TsFFwFcbgNM; Maurice Weaver, "Jerusalem Park Named after British Lung Donor," July 27, 2000, accessed November 17, 2010, http://www.telegraph.co.uk/news/worldnews/middleeast/israel/1350604/Jerusalem-park-named-after-British-lung-donor.html.

10. William Lamb, "Franklin Lakes Diabetes Patient Gets Gift of Life from a Stranger," November 7, 2010, accessed November 18, 2010, http://www.northjersey.com/news/106843628_From_a_stranger__the_gift_of_life.html.

11. Kathleen Ellis, "MUSC Student Gives Gift of Life to Stranger," August 21, 2009, accessed November 17, 20010, http://newsroom.muschealth.com/index.php/2009/08/musc-student-gives-gift-of-life-to-stranger.

12. Ibid.

13. Jennifer Bails, "Pay It Forward," *Carnegie Mellon Today*, January 2008, accessed November 18, 2010, http://www.carnegiemellontoday.com/article.asp?aid=514.

14. Ibid.

15. Thomas P. Genovese, "2010 Senior Inspiration Awards Nomination Form (Attachment 4)," January 5, 2010, accessed November 18, 2010, http://www.la-quinta.org/Modules/ShowDocument.aspx?documentid=9219.

16. Kenny Goldberg, "Altruistic Organ Donors Give to Perfect Strangers," March 18, 2010, accessed November 18, 2010, http://www.kpbs.org/news/2010/mar/18/altruistic-organ-donors-give-perfect-strangers.

17. Martha J. Morelock, "Giftedness: The View from Within," *Understanding Our Gifted* 4, no. 3 (1992): 14.

18. Jan Brunt, "Caring Thinking: The New Intelligence," *Gifted* 130 (2003): 13–14.
19. Ibid., 14–16.
20. Ibid., 15.

CHAPTER 15: CYNTHIA

1. Beth Saulnier, "The Strongest Link," *Cornell Alumni Magazine*, November 13, 2008, accessed December 15, 2010, http://cornellalumnimagazine.com/index.php?option=com_content&task=view&id=266.
2. Cynthia Marshall, interviewed by Rena Down, August 14, 2009.
3. Ibid., note 1.
4. National Kidney Registry, "Kidney Transplant Chain Initiated at New York-Presbyterian/Weill Cornell," February 20, 2008, accessed December 16, 2010, http://www.kidneyregistry.org/pages/p67/NYPres_Chain22008.php.
5. Marshall, interview by Down, August 14, 2009.
6. Ibid.
7. Ibid.
8. Ibid.
9. Ibid.

CHAPTER 16: KEN

1. Ken Schuler, telephone interview with Katrina Bramstedt, January 31, 2010.
2. Ken Schuler, "Welcome to the Black & White World of Pencil Drawings & Prints," accessed December 18, 2010, http://www.kenschuler.com.
3. Schuler, interview with Bramstedt, January 31, 2010.
4. Ibid.
5. Don Colburn, "Giving Organs: — You Don't Have to Be Dead — Or Even Related," *Seattle Times*, July 28, 1999, accessed December 16, 2010, http://community.seattletimes.nwsource.com/archive/?date=19990728&slug=2974072.
6. Schuler, interview with Bramstedt, January 31, 2010.
7. United Network for Organ Sharing, "Virginian Gives Liver to Stranger," August 20, 1999, accessed January 29, 2010, http://www.unos.org/news/newsDetail.asp?id=198.
8. Ibid.
9. Schuler, interview with Bramstedt, January 31, 2010.
10. Ibid.
11. Ibid.
12. Meg Gatto, "Liver Recipient Dies," February 18, 2007, accessed December 17, 2010, http://www.whsv.com/news/headlines/5917741.html.
13. Schuler, interview with Bramstedt, January 31, 2010.

CHAPTER 17: KAREN

1. Karen Ormiston, telephone interview with Rena Down, August 26, 2009.
2. Ibid.

CHAPTER 18: ALTRUISM, ABUNDANCE, AND SUFFERING

1. Ervin Staub, *The Psychology of Good and Evil: Why Children, Adults, and Groups Help and Harm Others* (Cambridge: Cambridge University Press, 2003), 446.
2. Samuel P. Oliner and Pearl M. Oliner, *The Altruistic Personality: Rescuers of Jews in Nazi Europe* (New York: Free Press, 1988).
3. Stuart B. Kleinman, "A Terrorist Hijacking: Victims' Experiences Initially and 9 Years Later," *Journal of Traumatic Stress* 2 (1989): 49–58.
4. Krzysztof Kaniasty and F. Norris, "Mobilization and Deterioration of Social Support Following Natural Disasters," *Current Directions in Psychological Science* 4, no. 3 (1995): 94–98.
5. Frances K. Grossman, Lynn Sorsoli, and Maryam Kia-Keating, "A Gale Force Wind: Meaning Making by Male Survivors of Childhood Sexual Abuse," *American Journal of Orthopsychiatry* 76, no. 4 (2006): 434–43.
6. J. Curtis McMillen and Cynthia Loveland Cook, "The Positive By-Products of Spinal Cord Injury and Their Correlates," *Rehabilitation Psychology* 48, no. 2 (2003): 77–85.
7. Yunqing Li, "Recovering from Spousal Bereavement in Later Life: Does Volunteer Participation Play a Role?," *Journal of Gerontology: Social Sciences* 62B, no. 4 (2007): S257–66.

CHAPTER 19: CHAD

1. Church of Jesus Christ of Latter Day Saints, "Humanitarian Efforts," accessed December 17, 2010, http://www.ldschurchnews.com/humanitarian.
2. Chad Hancey, telephone interview with Katrina Bramstedt, February 4, 2010.
3. Ibid.
4. Ibid.
5. UR Advocate4Life, "Significant Loved Ones of Living Heroes," accessed December 17, 2010, http://uradvocate4life.comxa.com/index.php?p=1_4.
6. In the United States, there are thousands of patients with organ failure who have posted their need for an organ transplant on personal or commercial websites. The two most common commercial sites are Craigslist.com and MatchingDonors.com.
7. Hancey, interview with Bramstedt, February 4, 2010.
8. Chad Hancey, "Stories about Living Donation: Nondirected Living Donation," accessed December 17, 2010, http://www.kidney.org/transplantation/livingdonors/shareShowStory.cfm?storyID=265.

9. Chad Hancey, "Dear Transplant Nurse," accessed December 17, 2010, http://www.trioweb.org/Nurses/TYHancey.pdf.

10. Chad Hancey, "TransplantBuddies.org Forums » Living Organ Donor Heroes » Altruistic Donation Message Board," December 7, 2009, accessed December 18, 2010, http://www.transplantbuddies.org/tbx/messages/9/82470.html?1265239461.

11. Ibid., note 5.

12. Chad Hancey, "Steve Baum's Blog & Such: Give the Gift of Life," April 1, 2010, accessed December 18, 2010, http://stevebaum.wordpress.com/whats-news.

13. Chad Hancey, "TransplantBuddies.org Forums » Living Organ Donor Heroes » Altruistic Donation Message Board," April 3, 2009, accessed December 18, 2010, http://www.transplantbuddies.org/tbx/messages/9/45690.html?1238788715.

CHAPTER 20: CURT

1. Curt Bludworth, interview by Katrina Bramstedt, California Pacific Medical Center Library, March 15, 2010.

2. Helena Oliviero, "What Ever Happened to . . . the Man Who Donated Half of His Liver?," *Atlanta Journal-Constitution*, December 22, 2008, accessed December 4, 2010, http://www.ajc.com/hotjobs/content/metro/atlanta/stories/2008/12/22/Curt_Bludworth_whatever.html.

3. Bludworth, interview by Bramstedt, March 15, 2010.

4. Ibid.

5. Ibid.

6. Ibid.

7. Ibid.

8. Ibid.

9. Ibid.

10. Oliviero, "What Ever Happened to . . ."

CHAPTER 21: GARRETT

1. "Man Used Shock Collar to Punish His Children," January 30, 2009, accessed December 22, 2010, http://www.whiotv.com/news/18605994/detail.html.

2. *State of Ohio v. Kurt D. Burg*, C.A. Case No. O4CA94, Court of Appeals of Ohio, Second Appellate District, Greene County, 2005 Ohio 3666; 2005 Ohio App. Lexis 3389, July 15, 2005.

3. Scott Patsko, "The Gift of a Better Life," *The Morning Journal*, May 8, 2005, accessed November 29, 2010, http://www.morningjournal.com/articles/2005/05/08/top%20stories/14489704.txt.

4. Garrett Gall, telephone interview with Rena Down, October 4, 2009.

5. Ibid.

6. Ibid.

7. Rie Akaho et al., "Bone Marrow Transplantation in Subjects with Mental Disorders," *Psychiatry and Clinical Neurosciences* 57, no. 3 (2003): 314.

8. Gall, interview with Down, October 4, 2009.

9. Ibid.

10. Patsko, "The Gift of a Better Life."

11. Gall, interview with Down, October 4, 2009.

CHAPTER 22: CANDIDACY EVALUATION

1. Cheryl Brennan, telephone interview with Katrina Bramstedt, January 23, 2010.

2. Kenny Goldberg, "Altruistic Organ Donors Give to Perfect Strangers," March 18, 2010, accessed November 18, 2010, http://www.kpbs.org/news/2010/mar/18/altruistic-organ-donors-give-perfect-strangers; Bonnie Estridge, "Meet the Man Who Became a Kidney Donor at 73 to Save the Life of His Nephew," *Mail Online*, January 10, 2010, accessed November 30, 2010, http://www.dailymail.co.uk/health/article-1241916/Meet-man-kidney-donor-73-save-life-nephew.html#ixzz16spb8J4w; Liz Hull, "Mother, 81, Becomes Oldest Living Kidney Donor with a Gift of Life to Her Son," *Mail Online*, April 30, 2008, accessed December 1, 2010, http://www.dailymail.co.uk/news/article-563037/Mother-81-oldest-living-kidney-donor-gift-life-son.html#ixzz16szTkPxm.

3. Katrina A. Bramstedt, "Probing Transplant and Living Donor Candidates about Their Participation in Organ Vending," *Progress in Transplantation* 20, no. 3 (2010): 293.

4. Ibid.

5. Mark L. Barr et al., "A Report of the Vancouver Forum on the Care of the Live Organ Donor: Lung, Liver, Pancreas, and Intestine Data and Medical Guidelines," *Transplantation* 81, no. 10 (2006): 1373–85.

6. A. V. Reisaeter et al., "Pregnancy and Birth after Kidney Donation: The Norwegian Experience," *American Journal of Transplantation* 9, no. 4 (2009): 820–24.

7. H. N. Ibrahim et al., "Pregnancy Outcomes after Kidney Donation," *American Journal of Transplantation* 9, no. 4 (2009): 825–34.

8. Ibid., 829.

9. Reisaeter et al., "Pregnancy and Birth."

10. Ibrahim et al. "Pregnancy Outcomes."

11. Ibid., 832.

12. Ann Young et al., "Discovering Misattributed Paternity in Living Kidney Donation: Prevalence, Preference, and Practice," *Transplantation* 87, no. 10 (2009): 1433.

13. 42 CFR 482.98(d) (2009).

CHAPTER 23: THE DONOR'S FAMILY CIRCLE

1. John Donne, *Devotions upon Emergent Occasions and Seuerall Steps in My Sicknes— Meditation XVII* (London: Printed by A. M. for Thomas Jones, 1624), 108.

2. Ian Parker, "The Gift: Zell Kravinsky Gave Away Millions: But Somehow It Wasn't Enough," *The New Yorker*, August 2, 2004, 54–63.

3. Ibid., 58.

4. Cheryl L. Jacobs et al., "Evolution of a Nondirected Kidney Donor Program: Lessons Learned," *Clinical Transplants* (2003): 283–91; Cheryl L. Jacobs et al., "Twenty-Two Nondirected Kidney Donors: An Update on a Single Center's Experience," *American Journal of Transplantation* 4, no. 7 (2004): 1110–16.

5. Sarah Clarke et al., "Insurance Issues in Living Kidney Donation," *Transplantation* 76, no. 6 (2003): 1008–9.

6. Robert Yang et al., "Insurability of Living Organ Donors: A Systematic Review," *American Journal of Transplantation* 7, no. 6 (2007): 1542–51.

7. South East Organ Procurement Foundation, "Initiative Will Track and Protect Health Status of Living Kidney Donors in U.S.A.," accessed January 14, 2011, http://www.seopf.org/lodn_info.htm.

8. "Health Care Living Will," Katrina A. Bramstedt, accessed November 1, 2010, http://www.transplantethics.com/livingwilladvdirective.html.

9. B. K. Lam et al., "Marital Adjustment after Interspouse Living Donor Liver Transplantation," *Transplantation Proceedings* 32, no. 7 (2000): 2095–96.

10. Roberta G. Simmons et al., *The Gift of Life: The Effect of Organ Transplantation on Individuals, Family and Societal Dynamics*, 2nd ed. (New Brunswick, NJ: Transaction Books, 1987), 293–300.

11. Shulchan Aruch Yoreh De'ah 251: 3.

12. "iHEARTGUTS," accessed November 2, 2010, http://iheartguts.com.

13. Channing Bete Company, *Anita's Second Chance—A Story about Organ and Tissue Donation: A Coloring & Activities Book* (South Deerfield, MA: Channing Bete Company, 1995).

CHAPTER 24: ORGAN DONATION SURGERY

1. Christoph Troppmann, "Living Donor Nephrectomy Techniques: Comparative Review and Critical Appraisal," in *Living Donor Organ Transplantation*, ed. Rainer W. G. Gruessner and Enrico Benedetti (New York: McGraw-Hill, 2008), 194–97.

2. Dilip Moonka, Sammy Saab, and James Trotter, *Living Donor Liver Transplantation* (Mount Laurel, NJ: American Society for Transplantation, 2007), 4.

3. "The Procedure: Lung," American Society for Transplantation, accessed October 14, 2010, http://www.healthy-donor.com/the_procedure/lung.aspx.

4. M. L. Barr et al., "Living Donor Lobar Lung Transplantation: Current Status and Future Directions," *Transplant Proceedings* 37, no. 9 (2005): 3983.

5. "The Procedure: Intestine," American Society for Transplantation, accessed October 14, 2010, http://www.healthy-donor.com/the_procedure/intesting.aspx; "The Procedure: Pancreas," American Society for Transplantation, accessed October 14, 2010, http://www.healthy-donor.com/the_procedure/pancreas.aspx.

6. "Steps of Bone Marrow or PBSC Donation," National Marrow Donor Program, accessed October 15, 2010, http://www.marrow.org/DONOR/When_You_re_Asked_to_Donate_fo/Steps_of_Donation/index.html.

7. M. Y. Lind et al., "Body Image after Laparoscopic or Open Donor Nephrectomy," *Surgical Endoscopy* 18, no. 8 (2004): 1276–79.

8. Derek A. DuBay et al., "Cosmesis and Body Image after Adult Right Lobe Living Liver Donation," *Transplantation* 89, no. 10 (2010): 1270–75.

CHAPTER 25: COMPLICATIONS

1. "Living Donor Buddies™," International Association of Living Donors, accessed October 13, 2010, http://www.livingdonorsonline.org.

2. U.S. Department of Health and Human Services Organ Procurement and Transplant Network Organ Distribution Policy 3.5.11.6, "Donation Status," United Network for Organ Sharing, November 9, 2010, accessed January 14, 2011, http://optn.transplant.hrsa.gov/policiesAndBylaws/policies.asp.

3. Hassan N. Ibrahim et al., "Long-Term Consequences of Kidney Donation," *New England Journal of Medicine* 360, no. 5 (2009): 459.

4. Dorry L. Segev et al., "Perioperative Mortality and Long-Term Survival Following Live Kidney Donation," *Journal of the American Medical Association* 303, no. 10 (2010): 959–66.

5. Amy L. Friedman et al., "Early Clinical and Economic Outcomes of Patients Undergoing Living Donor Nephrectomy in the United States," *Archives of Surgery* 145, no. 4 (2010): 356–62.

6. Bhargav Mistry et al., "World's Oldest Donor-Recipient Solid Organ Transplant?," *Dialysis & Transplantation* 39, no. 12 (2010): 534–35.

7. David A. Duchene et al., "Successful Outcomes of Older Donors in Laparoscopic Donor Nephrectomy," *Journal of Endourology* 24, no. 10 (2010): 1593.

8. Stephen C. Jacobs et al., "Laparoscopic Kidney Donation from Patients Older Than 60 Years," *Journal of the American College of Surgeons* 198, no. 6 (2004): 892.

9. United Network for Organ Sharing, "Living Donation: Information You Need to Know," 2009, p. 7, accessed October 14, 2010, http://www.transplantliving.org/SharedContentDocuments/Living_Donation_Booklet_Final.pdf.

10. U.S. Department of Health and Human Services Advisory Committee on Organ Transplantation, "Living Liver Donor Informed Consent for Evaluation," U.S. Department of Health and Human Services, accessed October 13, 2010, http://www.organdonor.gov/research/acotapp2.htm.

11. Taku Iida et al., "Surgery-Related Morbidity in Living Donors for Liver Transplantation," *Transplantation* 89, no. 10 (2010): 1276–82; Rafik M. Ghobrial et al., "Donor Morbidity after Living Donation for Liver Transplantation," *Gastroenterology* 135, no. 2 (2008): 468–76.

12. "Becoming a Living Donor: Lung," American Society of Transplantation, accessed October 13, 2010, http://www.healthy-donor.com/becoming_a_living_donor/lung.aspx.

13. Kathryn Flynn, "Live Donor Program," Second Wind Lung Transplant Association, accessed October 13, 2010, http://www.2ndwind.org/donor_program/livedonor.htm.

14. United Network for Organ Sharing Living Donor Committee, toll-free phone number in the United States: 888-894-6361; mailing address: PO Box 2484, Richmond, VA 23218, USA.

15. "Becoming a Living Donor," American Society of Transplantation, accessed October 13, 2010, http://www.healthy-donor.com/becoming_a_living_donor/default.aspx.

16. "Be The Match," National Marrow Donor Program, accessed October 13, 2010, http://www.marrow.org.

17. E. K. Massey et al., "Encouraging Psychological Outcomes after Altruistic Donation to a Stranger," *American Journal of Transplantation* 20, no. 6 (2010): 1448.

18. T. W. Reichman et al., "Anonymous Living Liver Donation: Donor Profiles and Outcomes," *American Journal of Transplantation* 10, no. 9 (2010): 2099.

19. Public Law 103-329, Section 629a. Treasury, Postal Service and General Government Appropriations Act, 1995, "Absence in connection with serving as a bone-marrow or organ donor."

20. "Living Donor Assistance Program," National Living Donor Assistance Center, accessed October 13, 2010, http://www.livingdonorassistance.org.

21. Barbara Thomas, "Heal with Love Foundation," accessed November 26, 2010, http://www.healwithlovefoundation.org/index.html.

CHAPTER 26: KEVIN

1. Kevin Gosling, telephone interview with Katrina Bramstedt, February 15, 2010.

2. Linda Wright et al., "Living Anonymous Liver Donation: Case Report and Ethical Justification," *American Journal of Transplantation* 7, no. 4 (2007): 1032–35.

3. Megan Ogilvie, "Man Donates Part of His Liver to Stranger," *Toronto Star*, December 10, 2010, accessed December 11, 2010, http://www.thestar.com/article/905408--man-donates-part-of-his-liver-to-stranger.

4. Gosling, interview with Bramstedt, February 15, 2010.

5. Ibid.

6. Ibid.

7. Sarah Green, "He Felt 'Blessed' to Donate Liver: Canada's First Anonymous Transplant of Its Type," *Toronto Sun*, April 21, 2006, accessed December 14, 2010, http://cnews.canoe.ca/CNEWS/Features/2006/04/21/1544066-sun.html.

8. Trillium Gift of Life Network, "Program for Reimbursing Expenses of Living Organ Donors (PRELOD)," accessed December 13, 2010, http://www.giftoflife.on.ca/page.cfm?id=23428851-405B-41D2-A9A9-9275EA6C78E7.

9. Gosling, interview with Bramstedt, February 15, 2010.

CHAPTER 27: CLAUDE

1. Jean-Bernard Otte, "Good Samaritan Liver Donor in Pediatric Transplantation," *Pediatric Transplantation* 13, no. 2 (2009): 155–59.

2. The identity of this donor is anonymized per the requirement of his donation, but he gave permission for the use of his first name. He was telephonically interviewed by Katrina Bramstedt on February 7, 2010.

3. Jochem Hoyer, "A Nondirected Kidney Donation and Its Consequences: Personal Experience of a Transplant Surgeon," *Transplantation* 76, no. 8 (2003): 1264–65.

4. "Euroliver Foundation," accessed December 7, 2010, http://www.euroliver.be.

5. Claude, interview by Bramstedt, February 7, 2010.

CHAPTER 28: THE ORGAN RECIPIENT: ETHICAL CONSIDERATIONS

1. Jeff Moyer, telephone interview with Katrina Bramstedt, July 28, 2010.

2. Debbie Council, "Resident Donates Kidney to Stranger," July 12, 2010, accessed November 24, 2010, http://donatelife-organdonation.blogspot.com/2010/07/donate-life-organ-donation-awareness_9097.html.

3. Nicole Lanstrum, telephone interview with Rena Down, August 10, 2009.

4. The identity of this donor is anonymized in this instance so as to not alarm the recipient. This interview was conducted telephonically by Rena Down on August 15, 2009.

5. Ibid.

6. The identity of this donor is anonymized in this instance so as to not implicate the transplant hospital. The interview was conducted telephonically by Katrina Bramstedt on January 21, 2010.

7. The identity of this donor is anonymized in this instance per the requirement of his donation. The interview was conducted telephonically by Katrina Bramstedt on February 7, 2010.

8. National Kidney Foundation, "Saying Thank You," accessed November 26, 2010, http://www.kidney.org/transplantation/livingDonors/honoringThnx.cfm.

9. Fred Brown, telephone interview with Katrina Bramstedt, January 30, 2010.

10. Ibid.

11. Ibid.

12. Ibid.

13. The identity of this donor is anonymized in this instance so as to protect the privacy of the recipient's spouse. The interview was conducted telephonically by Katrina Bramstedt on January 23, 2010.

14. Ibid.

15. Max Zapata, telephone interview with Katrina Bramstedt, February 6, 2010.

16. Ibid.

17. Barbara Anderson, "Kidney Donation Spurs 20 More," *Modesto Bee*, July 4, 2010, accessed November 26, 2010, http://www.modbee.com/2010/07/04/1238519/kidney-donation-spurs-20-more.html.

18. U.S. Department of Health and Human Services, Health Resources and Services Administration, Healthcare Systems Bureau, Division of Transplantation, *2009*

Annual Report of the U.S. Organ Procurement and Transplantation Network and the Scientific Registry of Transplant Recipients: Transplant Data 1999–2008, table 5.13d, Adjusted Patient Survival by Year of Transplant at 3 Months, 1 Year, 3 Years, 5 Years and 10 Years Living Donor Kidney Transplants, accessed November 26, 2010, http://www.ustransplant.org/annual_reports/current/513d_ki.htm.

19. U.S. Department of Health and Human Services, Health Resources and Services Administration, Healthcare Systems Bureau, Division of Transplantation, *2009 Annual Report of the U.S. Organ Procurement and Transplantation Network and the Scientific Registry of Transplant Recipients: Transplant Data 1999–2008*, table 9.13b, Adjusted Patient Survival by Year of Transplant at 3 Months, 1 Year, 3 Years, 5 Years and 10 Years Living Donor Liver Transplants, accessed November 26, 2010, http://www.ustransplant.org/annual_reports/current/913b_li.htm.

20. R. N. Matin et al., "Melanoma in Organ Transplant Recipients: Clinicopathological Features and Outcome in 100 Cases," *American Journal of Transplantation* 8, no. 9 (2008): 1891–900.

21. Ibid.

22. D. Samuel and C. Feray, "Hepatitis Viruses and Liver Transplantation," *Journal of Gastroenterology and Hepatology* 12, no. 9–10 (1997): S335–41.

23. Jean-Charles Duclos-Vallee and Mylene Sebagh, "Recurrence of Autoimmune Disease, Primary Sclerosing Cholangitis, Primary Biliary Cirrhosis, and Autoimmune Hepatitis after Liver Transplantation," *Liver Transplantation* 15, no. 11 (2009): S25–34.

24. Ibid.

25. Ibid.

26. Karine Hadaya et al., "Early Relapse of Autoimmune Glomerulonephritis after Kidney Transplantation despite Antibody Induction and Triple-Drug-Based Immunosuppression," *Transplantation* 89, no. 6 (2010): 767–69.

27. Pornpimo Rianthavorn et al., "Noncompliance with Immunosuppressive Medications in Pediatric and Adolescent Patients Receiving Solid-Organ Transplants," *Transplantation* 77, no. 5 (2004): 778–82.

28. Ken Schuler, telephone interview with Katrina Bramstedt, January 31, 2010; Meredyth Censullo, "Meredyth's Blog for Monday, Feb. 19th," accessed November 29, 2010, http://www.wtsp.com/news/watercooler/story.aspx?storyid=49492.

29. Ibid.

30. Ibid.

31. Curt Bludworth, interview by Katrina Bramstedt, California Pacific Medical Center Library, March 15, 2010.

32. Dave Manglos, telephone interview with Katrina Bramstedt, February 1, 2010.

33. Brad Melekian, "Dozens Stage Ride to Honor Memory of Friend," May 5, 2008, *Union-Tribune*, accessed November 29, 2010, http://www.signonsandiego.com/sports/20080505-9999-1s5surfcol.html.

34. Garrett Gall, telephone interview with Rena Down, October 4, 2009.

35. Scott Patsko, "The Gift of a Better Life," *The Morning Journal*, May 8, 2005, accessed November 29, 2010, http://www.morningjournal.com/articles/2005/05/08/top%20stories/14489704.txt.

CHAPTER 29: LIFE AFTER DONATION

1. Mariana Lozada, Paola D'Adamo, and Miguel Angel Fuentes, "Rewarding Altruism," Santa Fe Institute Working Paper no. 10-07-014, July 21, 2010, accessed November 13, 2010, http://www.santafe.edu/media/workingpapers/10-07-014.pdf.

2. Thomas Baumgartner et al., "Oxytocin Shapes the Neural Circuitry of Trust and Trust Adaptation in Humans, *Neuron* 58, no. 4 (2008): 639–50.

3. Gregor Domes et al., "Oxytocin Improves 'Mind-Reading' in Humans," *Biological Psychiatry* 61, no. 6 (2007): 731–33.

4. Markus Heinrichs et al., "Social Support and Oxytocin Interact to Suppress Cortisol and Subjective Responses to Psychosocial Stress," *Biological Psychiatry* 54, no. 12 (2003): 1389–98.

5. Michael Kosfeld et al., "Oxytocin Increases Trust in Humans," *Nature* 435, no. 7042 (2005): 673–76.

6. Stephanie L. Brown et al., "Social Closeness Increases Salivary Progesterone in Humans," *Hormones and Behavior* 56, no. 1 (2009): 108–11; Stephanie L. Brown and R. Michael Brown, "Selective Investment Theory: Recasting the Functional Significance of Close Relationships," *Psychological Inquiry* 17, no. 1 (2006): 1–29.

7. Allan Luks and Peggy Payne, *The Healing Power of Doing Good* (Lincoln, NE: iUniverse.com, 2001), 10.

8. Ibid., 17.

9. Carolyn Schwartz et al., "Altruistic Social Interest Behaviors Are Associated with Better Mental Health," *Psychosomatic Medicine* 65, no. 5 (2003): 778–85.

10. Ibid., 782.

11. Jack Marschall, telephone interview with Rena Down, August 22, 2009.

12. Lori Palatnik, "PART 1 (of 4): Why I Donated a Kidney to a Total Stranger," accessed November 9, 2010, http://il.youtube.com.

13. Chaya Lipschutz, "Kidneymitzvah's Channel," accessed November 9, 2010, http://www.youtube.com/user/Kidneymitzvah#p/f.

14. Jean-Bernard Otte, "Good Samaritan Liver Donor in Pediatric Transplantation," *Pediatric Transplantation* 13, no. 2 (2009): 155–59.

15. Linda Wright et al., "Living Anonymous Liver Donation: Case Report and Ethical Justification," *American Journal of Transplantation* 7, no. 4 (2007): 1032–35.

16. Laura M. Prager et al., "Medical and Psychologic Outcome of Living Lobar Lung Transplant Donors," *Journal of Heart and Lung Transplantation* 25, no. 10 (2006): 1206–12.

17. Ibid., 1210.

18. Margareta A. Sanner, "The Donation Process of Living Kidney Donors," *Nephrology Dialysis Transplantation* 20 (2005): 1707–13.

19. Ibid., 1710.

20. The identity of this donor is anonymized in this instance because of the sensitivity of the topic.

21. Ibid.

22. Ibid.

23. Ibid.

24. Ibid.

25. Ibid.

26. Ibid.

27. Ibid., note 12.

28. Jeff Moyer, telephone interview with Katrina Bramstedt, July 28, 2010.

29. "Christian Kidney Foundation," accessed November 7, 2010, http://christian kidneyfoundation.org.

30. Arlene Arthur, interview by Katrina Bramstedt, California Pacific Medical Center Library, June 27, 2009.

31. Matthew Auchter, telephone interview with Rena Down, August 10, 2009.

32. "24th Annual Stair Climb to Cure Cystic Fibrosis March 12 at One America Plaza," *San Diego Metropolitan Magazine and Daily Business Report*, March 2005, accessed November 16, 2010, http://sandiegometro.archives.whsites.net/2005/mar/sdscene5.php.

33. Chad Hancey, telephone interview with Katrina Bramstedt, February 4, 2010.

34. Email communication from Scott Good to Katrina Bramstedt, February 13, 2011.

35. Ibid., note 31.

36. Ken Schuler, telephone interview with Katrina Bramstedt, January 31, 2010.

37. National Kidney Foundation, "Get Involved: Living Donors," accessed February 14, 2011, http://www.kidney.org/news/tgames2010/livingdonors/index.cfm.

38. World Transplant Games Federation, "World Transplant Games Federation," accessed February 14, 2011, http://www.wtgf.org/default.asp.

CHAPTER 30: ELEVATION

1. Allan Luks and Peggy Payne, *The Healing Power of Doing Good* (Lincoln, NE: iUniverse.com, 2001), 10.

2. Jonathan Haidt, "Elevation and the Positive Psychology of Morality," in *Flourishing: Positive Psychology and the Life Well-Lived*, ed. C. L. M. Keyes and Jonathan Haidt (Washington, DC: American Psychological Association, 2003), 281.

3. Jonathan Haidt, "Wired to Be Inspired," *Greater Good*, Spring/Summer 2005: 7–8.

4. Keith S. Cox, "Elevation Predicts Domain-Specific Volunteerism 3 Months Later," *Journal of Positive Psychology* 5, no. 5 (2010): 333.

5. Ibid., note 3, p. 8.

6. Sara B. Algoea and Jonathan Haidt, "Witnessing Excellence in Action: The 'Other-Praising' Emotions of Elevation, Gratitude, and Admiration," *Journal of Positive Psychology* 4, no. 2 (2009): 117–18.

7. Thomas Jefferson, letter to Robert Skipwith, in *The Portable Thomas Jefferson*, ed. M. D. Peterson (New York: Penguin, 1975), 349 (original work published August 3, 1771).

8. Ibid., 350.

9. Ibid., note 3, p. 8.

10. Ibid., note 4, pp. 333–41.

11. Ibid., note 3, page 7.

12. Ibid., note 4, pp. 333–41.

13. In the United States, adults and teenagers (in several states) can register their desire to donate organs on their death at their state motor vehicle registration bureau or their state donor registration website. For more information, go to http://www .donatelife.net (Donate Life America). In Canada, contact the Organ Donation and Transplant Association of Canada (http://organdonations.ca/help/organdonor).

14. Ibid., note 6.

Bibliography

Akaho, R., T. Sasaki, M. Yoshino, K. Hagiya, H. Akiyama, and H. Sakamaki. "Bone Marrow Transplantation in Subjects with Mental Disorders." *Psychiatry and Clinical Neurosciences* 57, no. 3 (2003): 311–15.

Algoea, Sara B., and Jonathan Haidt. "Witnessing Excellence in Action: the 'Other-Praising' Emotions of Elevation, Gratitude, and Admiration." *Journal of Positive Psychology* 4, no. 2 (2009): 105–27.

American Society of Transplantation. "Becoming a Living Donor." Accessed October 13, 2010. www.healthy-donor.com/becoming_a_living_donor/default.aspx.

American Society of Transplantation. "Becoming a Living Donor: Lung." Accessed October 13, 2010. www.healthy-donor.com/becoming_a_living_donor/lung.aspx.

American Society for Transplantation. "The Procedure: Intestine." Accessed October 14, 2010. www.healthy-donor.com/the_procedure/intesting.aspx.

American Society for Transplantation. "The Procedure: Lung." Accessed October 14, 2010. www.healthy-donor.com/the_procedure/lung.aspx.

American Society for Transplantation. "The Procedure: Pancreas." Accessed October 14, 2010. www.healthy-donor.com/the_procedure/pancreas.aspx.

Bails, Jennifer. "Pay it Forward." *Carnegie Mellon Today*, January 2008. Accessed November 18, 2010. www.carnegiemellontoday.com/article.asp?aid=514.

Barasch, Marc Ian. *Field Notes on a Compassionate Life: A Search for the Soul of Kindness.* Emmaus, PA: Rodale, 2005.

Barr, M. L., J. Belghiti, F. G. Villamil, E. A. Pomfret, D. S. Sutherland, R. W. Gruessnerm, A. N. Langnas, and F. L. Delmonico. "A Report of the Vancouver Forum on the Care of the Live Organ Donor: Lung, Liver, Pancreas, and Intestine Data and Medical Guidelines." *Transplantation* 81, no. 10 (2006): 1373–85.

Barr, M. L., F. A. Schenkel, M. E. Bowdish, and V. A. Starnes. "Living Donor Lobar Lung Transplantation: Current Status and Future Directions." *Transplant Proceedings* 37, no. 9 (2005): 3983–86.

Baumgartner T., M. Heinrichs, A. Vonlanthen, U. Fischbacher, and E. Fehr. "Oxytocin Shapes the Neural Circuitry of Trust and Trust Adaptation in Humans." *Neuron* 58, no.4 (2008): 639–50.

Bayne, T., and Neil Levy. "Amputees by Choice: Body Integrity Identity Disorder and the Ethics of Amputation." *Journal of Applied Philosophy* 22, no.1 (2005): 75–86.

Bordereau, C., A. Robert, V. Van Tuyen, and A. Peppuy. "Suicidal Defensive Behaviour by Frontal Gland Dehiscence in Globitermes sulphureus Haviland Soldiers (Isoptera)." *Insectes Sociaux* 44, no. 3 (1997): 289–96.

Bramstedt, Katrina A. "Probing Transplant and Living Donor Candidates About Their Participation in Organ Vending." *Progress in Transplantation* 20, no. 3 (2010): 292–95.

Brown, S. L., B. L. Fredrickson, M. M. Wirth, M. J. Poulin, E. A. Meier, E. D. Heaphy, M. D. Cohen, and O. C. Schultheiss. "Social Closeness Increases Salivary Progesterone in Humans." *Hormones and Behavior* 56, no.1 (2009): 108–11.

Brown, S. L., and R. Michael Brown. "Selective Investment Theory: Recasting the Functional Significance of Close Relationships." *Psychological Inquiry* 17, no. 1 (2006): 1–29.

Brunt, Jan. "Caring Thinking: The New Intelligence." *Gifted* 130 (2003): 13–16.

Channing Bete Company. *Anita's Second Chance—A Story About Organ and Tissue Donation: A Coloring & Activities Book.* South Deerfield, MA: Channing Bete Company, 1995.

Clarke, Sarah, J. A. Lumsdaine, S. J. Wigmore, M. Akyol, and J. L. Forsythe. "Insurance Issues in Living Kidney Donation." *Transplantation* 76, no. 6 (2003): 1008–9.

Condition of Participation: Human Resources, *Code of Federal Regulations* Title 42, Chapter IV, §482.98(d), October 1, 2009.

Connor, Richard C., and Kenneth S. Norris. "Are Dolphins Reciprocal Altruists?" *American Naturalist* 199, no. 3 (1982): 358–74.

Cox, Keith S. "Elevation Predicts Domain-Specific Volunteerism 3 Months Later." *Journal of Positive Psychology* 5, no. 5 (2010): 333–41.

Davis, M. H. "Measuring Individual Differences in Empathy: Evidence for a Multidimensional Approach." *Journal of Personality and Social Psychology* 44, no. 1 (1983): 113–24.

Department of Treasury and General Government Appropriations Act of 1995, Public Law 103–329, Section 629a (1995).

Dixon, D. J., and S. E. Abbey. "Religious Altruism and the Living Organ Donor." *Progress in Transplantation* 13, no. 3 (2003): 169–75.

Domes G., M. Heinrichs, A. Michel, C. Berger, and S. C. Herpertz. "Oxytocin Improves 'Mind-Reading' in Humans." *Biological Psychiatry* 61, no. 6 (2007): 731–33.

DuBay, D. A., S. Holtzman, L. Adcock, S. E. Abbey, S. Greenwood, C. Macleod, A. Kashfi, E. L. Renner, D. R. Grant, G. A. Levy, and G. Therapondos. "Cosmesis and Body Image After Adult Right Lobe Living Liver Donation." *Transplantation* 89, no. 10 (2010): 1270–75.

Duchene, D. A., D. Y. Woodruff, B. L. Gallagher, H. A. Aubert, D. Katz, T. B. Dunn, and H. N. Winfield. "Successful Outcomes of Older Donors in Laparoscopic Donor Nephrectomy." *Journal of Endourology* 24, no. 10 (2010): 1593–96.

Duclos-Vallee, J. C., and Mylene Sebagh. "Recurrence of Autoimmune Disease, Primary Sclerosing Cholangitis, Primary Biliary Cirrhosis, and Autoimmune Hepatitis After Liver Transplantation." *Liver Transplantation* 15, no. 11 (2009): S25–S34.

Esmond, J., and P. Dunlop. *Developing the Volunteer Motivation Inventory to Assess the Underlying Motivational Drives of Volunteers in Western Australia.* 2004. Accessed September 1, 2010. www.mtd4u.com/resources/MotivationFinalReport.pdf.

Estridge, Bonnie. "Meet the Man Who Became a Kidney Donor at 73 to Save the Life of His Nephew." *Mail Online*, January 10, 2010. Accessed November 30, 2010. www.dailymail.co.uk/health/article-1241916/Meet-man-kidney-donor-73-save -life-nephew.html#ixzz16spb8J4w.

Friedman, A. L., K. Cheung K, S. A. Roman, and J. A. Sosa. "Early Clinical and Economic Outcomes of Patients Undergoing Living Donor Nephrectomy in the United States." *Archives of Surgery* 145, no. 4 (2010): 356–62.

Ghobrial, R. M., C. E. Freise, J. F. Trotter, L. Tong, A. O. Ojo, J. H. Fair, R. A. Fisher, J. C. Emond, A. J. Koffron, T. L. Pruett, K. M. Olthoff; A2ALL Study Group. "Donor Morbidity After Living Donation for Liver Transplantation." *Gastroenterology* 135, no.2 (2008): 468–76.

Gohh, R. Y., P. E. Morrissey, P. N. Madras, and A. P. Monaco. "Controversies in Organ Donation: The Altruistic Living Donor." *Nephrology, Dialysis, Transplantation* 16, no. 3 (2001): 619–21.

Green, Sarah. "He Felt 'Blessed' to Donate Liver: Canada's First Anonymous Transplant of Its Type." *Toronto Sun*, April 21, 2006. Accessed December 14, 2010. www.cnews.canoe.ca/CNEWS/Features/2006/04/21/1544066-sun.html.

Grossman, Frances K., Lynn Sorsoli, and Maryam Kia-Keating. "A Gale Force Wind: Meaning Making by Male Survivors of Childhood Sexual Abuse." *American Journal of Orthopsychiatry* 76, no. 4 (2006): 434–43.

Hadaya, K., N. Marangon, S. Moll, S. Ferrari-Lacraz, and J. Villard. "Early Relapse of Autoimmune Glomerulonephritis After Kidney Transplantation Despite Antibody Induction and Triple-Drug-Based Immunosuppression." *Transplantation* 89, no. 6 (2010): 767-69.

Haidt, Jonathan. "Elevation and the Positive Psychology of Morality." In *Flourishing: Positive Psychology and the Life Well-Lived*, edited by C.L.M. Keyes and Jonathan Haidt, 275–89. Washington DC: American Psychological Association, 2003.

Haidt, Jonathan. "Wired to Be Inspired." *Greater Good* Spring/Summer 2005: 6–9.

Heinrichs, Markus, T. Baumgartner, C. Kirschbaum, and U. Ehlert. "Social Support and Oxytocin Interact to Suppress Cortisol and Subjective Responses to Psychosocial Stress." *Biological Psychiatry* 54, no. 12 (2003): 1389–98.

Henderson, A. J., M. A. Landolt, M. F. McDonald, W. M. Barrable, J. G. Soos, W. Gourlay, C. J. Allison, and D. N. Landsberg. "The Living Anonymous Kidney Donor: Lunatic or Saint?" *American Journal of Transplantation* 3, no. 2 (2003): 203–13.

Hoyer, Jochem. "A Nondirected Kidney Donation and Its Consequences: Personal Experience of a Transplant Surgeon." *Transplantation* 76, no. 8 (2003):1264–65.

Hull, Liz. "Mother, 81, Becomes Oldest Living Kidney Donor with a Gift of Life to Her Son." *Mail Online*, April 30, 2008. Accessed December 1, 2010. www

.dailymail.co.uk/news/article-563037/Mother-81-oldest-living-kidney-donor-gift
-life-son.html#ixzz16szTkPxm.

Ibrahim, H. N., R. Foley, L. Tan, T. Rogers, R. F. Bailey, H. Guo, C. R. Gross, and
A. J. Matas. "Long-Term Consequences of Kidney Donation." *New England Journal
of Medicine* 360, no. 5 (2009): 459–69.

Ibrahim, H. N., S. K. Akkina, E. Leister, K. Gillingham, G. Cordner, H. Guo,
R. Bailey, T. Rogers, and A. J. Matas. "Pregnancy Outcomes After Kidney Donation." *American Journal of Transplantation* 9, no. 4 (2009): 825–34.

Iida, T., Y. Ogura, F. Oike, E. Hatano, T. Kaido, H. Egawa, Y. Takada, and S. Ue-
moto. "Surgery-Related Morbidity in Living Donors for Liver Transplantation."
Transplantation 89, no. 10 (2010): 1276–82.

International Association of Living Donors. "Living Donor Buddies™." Accessed
October 13, 2010. www.livingdonorsonline.org.

Jacobs, Cheryl L., C. Garvey, D. Roman, J. Kahn, and A. J. Matas. "Evolution of a
Nondirected Kidney Donor Program: Lessons Learned." *Clinical Transplants* 2003:
283–91.

Jacobs, Cheryl L., D. Roman, C. Garvey, J. Kahn, and A. J. Matas. "Twenty-Two
Nondirected Kidney Donors: An Update on a Single Center's Experience." *American Journal of Transplantation* 4, no. 7 (2004): 1110–116.

Jacobs, S. C., J. R. Ramey, G. N. Sklar, and S. T. Bartlett. "Laparoscopic Kidney
Donation From Patients Older Than 60 Years." *Journal of the American College of
Surgeons* 198, no. 6 (2004): 892–97.

Jefferson, T. Letter to Robert Skipwith. *The Portable Thomas Jefferson*, edited by
M. D. Peterson, 349–50. New York: Penguin, 1975. (Original work published
August 3, 1771.)

Jendrisak, M. D., B. Hong, S. Shenoy, J. Lowell, N. Desai, W. Chapman, A. Vijayan,
R. D. Wetzel, M. Smith, J. Wagner, S. Brennan, D. Brockmeier, and D. Kappel.
"Altruistic Living Donors: Evaluation for Nondirected Kidney or Liver Donation."
American Journal of Transplantation 6, no. 1 (2006): 115–20.

Jesus Christians. "Kidneys." Accessed October 28, 2008. www.jesus-teachings.com/
kidneys.

Kaniasty, Krzyszt, and F. Norris. "Mobilization and Deterioration of Social Support Following Natural Disasters." *Current Directions in Psychological Science* 4, no. 3
(1995): 94–98.

Kleinman, Stuart B. "A Terrorist Hijacking: Victims' Experiences Initially and 9 Years
later." *Journal of Traumatic Stress* 2 (1989): 49–58.

Knafo, Ariel, and Robert Plomin. "Parental Discipline and Affection and Children's
Prosocial Behavior: Genetic and Environmental Links." *Journal of Personality and
Social Psychology* 90, no. 1 (2006): 147–64.

Kohlberg, Lawrence. "Moral Stages and Moralization: The Cognitive-Developmental
Approach." *Moral Development and Behavior: Theory, Research, and Social Issues*, edited
by Tom Lickona, 31–53. New York: Holt, Rinehart & Winston, 1976.

Kosfeld, M., M. Heinrichs, P. J. Zak, U. Fischbacher, and E. Fehr. "Oxytocin Increases Trust in Humans." *Nature* 435, no. 7042 (2005): 673–76.

Lam, B. K. C. M. Lo, A. S. Fung, S. T. Fan, C. L. Liu, and J. Wong. "Marital Adjustment After Interspouse Living Donor Liver Transplantation," *Transplantation Proceedings* 32, no. 7 (2000): 2095–96.

Lavelle, Janet. "San Diego Couple Final Link in Kidney Transplant Chain." *San Diego Union-Tribune*, August 28, 2010. Accessed October 28, 2010. www.signonsandiego .com/news/2010/aug/27/san-diego-couple-participates-nations-largest-kidn/

Li, Yunquing. "Recovering From Spousal Bereavement in Later Life: Does Volunteer Participation Play a Role?" *Journal of Gerontology: Social Sciences* 62B, no. 4 (2007): S257–66.

Lind, M.Y., W. C. Hop, W. Weimar, and J. N. IJzermans. "Body Image After Laparoscopic or Open Donor Nephrectomy." *Surgical Endoscopy* 18, no. 8 (2004): 1276–79.

Lozada, Mariana, Paola D'Adamo, and Miguel Angel Fuentes. "Rewarding Altruism." Santa Fe Institute Working Paper #10-07-014, July 21, 2010. Accessed November 13, 2010. www.santafe.edu/media/workingpapers/10-07-014.pdf.

Luks, Allan, and Peggy Payne. *The Healing Power of Doing Good*. Lincoln, NE: iUniverse.com, 2001.

Massey, E. K., L. W. Kranenburg, W. C. Zuidema, G. Hak, R. A. Erdman, M. Hilhorst, J. N. Ijzermans, J. J. Busschbach, and W. Weimar. "Encouraging Psychological Outcomes After Altruistic Donation to a Stranger." *American Journal of Transplantation* 10, no. 6 (2010): 1445–52.

Mathur, V. A., T. Harada, T. Lipke, and J. Y. Chiao. "Neural Basis of Extraordinary Empathy and Altruistic Motivation." *NeuroImage* 51, no. 4 (2010): 1468–75.

Matin, R. N., D. Mesher, C. M. Proby, J. M. McGregor, J. N. Bouwes Bavinck, V. Del Marmol, S. Euvrard, C. Ferrandiz, A. Geusau, M. Hackethal, W. L. Ho, G. F. L. Hofbauer, B. Imko-Walczuk, J. Kanitakis, A. Lally, J. T. Lear, C. Lebbe, G. M. Murphy, S. Piaserico, D. Seckin, E. Stockfleth, C. Ulrich, F. T. Wojnarowska, H. Y. Lin, C. Balch, C. A. Harwood, on behalf of the Skin Care in Organ Transplant Patients, Europe (SCOPE) group. "Melanoma in Organ Transplant Recipients: Clinicopathological Features and Outcome in 100 Cases." *American Journal of Transplantation* 8, no. 9 (2008): 1891–900.

McMillen, J. C., and Cynthia Loveland Cook. "The Positive By-Products of Spinal Cord Injury and Their Correlates." *Rehabilitation Psychology* 48, no. 2 (2003): 77–85.

Melekian, Brad. "Dozens Stage Ride to Honor Memory of Friend." *Union-Tribune*, May 5, 2008. Accessed November 29, 2010. www.signonsandiego.com/sports/20080505-9999-1s5surfcol.html.

Merullo, Roland. "Every Breath He Takes." *Reader's Digest*, December 2003. Accessed December 8, 2010. www.rd.com/content/printContent.do?contentId=285 62&KeepThis=true&TB_iframe=true&height=500&width=790&modal=true.

Mistry, Bhargav, Brian McKeever, Gautam Phadke, and Adit Mahale. "World's Oldest Donor-Recipient Solid Organ Transplant?" *Dialysis & Transplantation* 39, no. 12 (2010): 534–35.

Moonka, Dilip, Sammy Saab, and James Trotter. *Living Donor Liver Transplantation*. Mount Laurel, NJ: American Society for Transplantation, 2007.

Morelock, Martha J. "Giftedness: The View From Within." *Understanding Our Gifted* 4, no. 3 (1992): 11–15.

Moyer, Jeff. "Giving a Kidney, Gaining a Lifelong Friend." *National Public Radio*, September 13, 2010. Accessed December 10, 2010. www.npr.org/templates/story/story.php?storyId=129731335.

Mueller, P. S., E. J. Case, and C. C. Hook. "Responding to Offers of Altruistic Living Unrelated Kidney Donation by Group Associations: An Ethical Analysis." *Transplantation Reviews* 22, no. 3 (2008): 200–205.

National Marrow Donor Program. "Be The Match." Accessed October 13, 2010 .www.marrow.org.

Nichols, Shaun. "Mindreading and the Cognitive Architecture Underlying Altruistic Motivation." *Mind & Language* 16 (2001): 425–55.

Nogueira, J. M., M. R. Weir, S. Jacobs, D. Breault, D. Klassen, D. A. Evans, S. T. Bartlett, and M. Cooper. "A Study of Renal Outcomes in Obese Living Kidney Donors." *Transplantation* 90, no. 9 (2010): 993–99.

Oliner, Samuel P., and Pearl M. Oliner. *The Altruistic Personality: Rescuers of Jews in Nazi Europe.* New York: Free Press, 1988.

Oliviero, Helena. "What Ever Happened to . . . The Man Who Donated Half of His Liver?" *Atlanta Journal-Constitution*, December 22, 2008. Accessed December 4, 2010. www.ajc.com/hotjobs/content/metro/atlanta/stories/2008/12/22/Curt_Bludworth_whatever.html.

Organ Donation, SB 1395, State of California (September 2, 2010).

Park, Jerry Z., and Christian Smith. "'To Whom Much Has Been Given...': Religious Capital and Community Voluntarism Among Churchgoing Protestants." *Journal for the Scientific Study of Religion* 39, no. 3 (2000): 272–86.

Parker, Ian. "The Gift: Zell Kravinsky Gave Away Millions: But Somehow It Wasn't Enough." *New Yorker*, August 2, 2004:54–63.

Patrone, Dan. "Disfigured Anatomies and Imperfect Analogies: Body Integrity Identity Disorder and the Supposed Right to Self-Demanded Amputation of Healthy Body Parts." *Journal of Medical Ethics* 35, no. 9 (2009): 541–45.

Patsko, Scott. "The Gift of a Better Life." *The Morning Journal*, May 8, 2005. Accessed November 29, 2010. www.morningjournal.com/articles/2005/05/08/top%20stories/14489704.txt.

Prager, L. M., J .C. Wain, D. H. Roberts, and L. C. Ginns. "Medical and Psychologic Outcome of Living Lobar Lung Transplant Donors." *Journal of Heart and Lung Transplantation* 25, no. 10 (2006): 1206–12.

Prohibition of Organ Purchases. Public Law 98-507, Title III, Section 301a (1984).

Reichman, T. W., A. Fox, L. Adcock, L. Wright, S. E. Abbey, G. Levy, and D. R. Grant. "Anonymous Living Liver Donation: Donor Profiles and Outcomes." *American Journal of Transplantation* 10, no. 9 (2010): 2099–2104.

Reisaeter, A. V., J. Røislien, T. Henriksen, L. M. Irgens, and A. Hartmann. "Pregnancy and Birth After Kidney Donation: The Norwegian Experience." *American Journal of Transplantation* 9, no. 4 (2009): 820–24.

Reuter, M., C. Frenzel, N. T. Walter, S. Markett, and C. Montag. "Investigating the Genetic Basis of Altruism: The Role of the COMT Val158Met Polymorphism." *Social Cognitive and Affective Neuroscience*, October 28, 2010 [Epub ahead of print].

Rianthavorn, P., R. B. Ettenger, M. Malekzadeh, J. L. Marik, M. Struber. "Noncompliance with Immunosuppressive Medications in Pediatric and Adolescent Patients Receiving Solid-Organ Transplants." *Transplantation* 77, no. 5 (2004): 778–82.

Rosenhan, David. "The Natural Socialization of Altruistic Autonomy." In *Altruism and Helping Behavior*, edited by Jacqueline Macaulay and Leonard Berkowitz, 251–68. New York: Academic Press, 1970.

Rueppell, O., M. K. Hayworth, and N. P. Ross. "Altruistic Self-Removal of Health-Compromised Honey Bee Workers From Their Hive." *Journal of Evolutional Biology* 23, no. 7 (2010): 1538–46.

Rushton, J. Philippe. "Is Altruism Innate?" *Psychological Inquiry* 2 (1991): 141–43.

Sadler, H. H., L. Davison, C. Carroll, and S. L. Kountz. "The Living, Genetically Unrelated, Kidney Donor." *Seminars in Psychiatry* 3, no. 1 (1971): 86–101.

Samuel, D., and C. Feray. "Hepatitis Viruses and Liver Transplantation." *Journal of Gastroenterology and Hepatology* 12, no. 9–10 (1997): S335–41.

Sanner, Margareta A. "The Donation Process of Living Kidney Donors." *Nephrology Dialysis Transplantation* 20, no. 8 (2005):1707–13.

Schneider, Keith. "Plane Crash in Georgia Kills 23, Including Former Senator Tower." *New York Times*, April 6, 1991. Accessed December 9, 2010. www .nytimes.com/1991/04/06/us/plane-crash-in-georgia-kills-23-including-former -senator-tower.html.

Schwartz, C., J. B. Meisenhelder, Y. Ma, and G. Reed. "Altruistic Social Interest Behaviors Are Associated with Better Mental Health." *Psychosomatic Medicine* 65, no. 5 (2003): 778–85.

Second Wind Lung Transplant Association. "Live Donor Program." Accessed October 13, 2010. www.2ndwind.org/donor_program/livedonor.htm.

Segev, D. L., A. D. Muzaale, B. S. Caffo, S. H. Mehta, A. L. Singer, S. E. Taranto, M. A. McBride, and R. A. Montgomery. "Perioperative Mortality and Long-Term Survival Following Live Kidney Donation." *Journal of the American Medical Association* 303, no. 10 (2010): 959–66.

Simmons R. G., Susan Klein Marine, and Richard L. Simmons. *The Gift of Life: The Effect of Organ Transplantation on Individuals, Family and Societal Dynamics*. 2nd ed. New Brunswick, NJ: Transaction Books, 1987.

Simpson, Martha. "If You Can't Donate" (unpublished manuscript), Raleigh, NC, November 13, 2006.

Staub, Ervin. "Helping a Distressed Person: Social, Personality, and Stimulus Determinants." *Advances in Experimental Social Psychology* 7 (1974): 293–41.

Staub, Ervin. *The Psychology of Good and Evil: Why Children, Adults, and Groups Help and Harm Others*. Cambridge: Cambridge University Press, 2003.

Troppmann, Christoph. "Living Donor Nephrectomy Techniques: Comparative Review and Critical Appraisal." In *Living Donor Organ Transplantation*, edited by Rainer W. G. Gruessner and Enrico Benedetti, 194–97. New York: McGraw-Hill, 2008.

United Network for Organ Sharing. *Living Donation: Information You Need to Know*. Richmond, VA: United Network for Organ Sharing, 2009. Accessed October 14, 2010. www.transplantliving.org/SharedContentDocuments/Living_Donation_ Booklet_Final.pdf.

US Department of Health and Human Services. Organ Procurement and Transplant Network Organ Distribution Policy 3.5.11.6, "Donation Status," United Network for Organ Sharing, November 9, 2010. Accessed January 14, 2011. www.optn .transplant.hrsa.gov/policiesAndBylaws/policies.asp.

US Department of Health and Human Services Advisory Committee on Organ Transplantation. "Living Liver Donor Informed Consent For Evaluation." Accessed October 13, 2010. www.organdonor.gov/research/acotapp2.htm.

US Department of Health and Human Services, Health Resources and Services Administration, Healthcare Systems Bureau, Division of Transplantation. *2009 Annual Report of the U.S. Organ Procurement and Transplantation Network and the Scientific Registry of Transplant Recipients: Transplant Data 1999-2008*, Rockville: MD, 2009.

Warneken, Felix, and Michael Tomasello. "The Roots of Human Altruism." *British Journal of Psychology* 100, Part 3 (2009): 455–71.

Whiting, Sam. "Transplant Ethicist Guards Organ Donors' Rights." *San Francisco Chronicle*, March 23, 2009. Accessed December 23, 2010. www.cpmc.org/advanced/ kidney/news/Bramstedt.pdf.

Wilson J., and M. Musick. *Volunteers: A Social Profile*. Bloomington: Indiana University Press, 2008.

Wright, Linda, K. Ross, S. Abbey, G. Levy, and D. Grant. "Living Anonymous Liver Donation: Case Report and Ethical Justification." *American Journal of Transplantation* 7, no. 4 (2007): 1032–35.

Young, A., S. J. Kim, E. M. Gibney, C. R. Parikh, M. S. Cuerden, L. D. Horvat, P. Hizo-Abes, and A. X. Garg; Donor Nephrectomy Outcomes Research (DONOR) Network. "Discovering Misattributed Paternity in Living Kidney Donation: Prevalence, Preference, and Practice." *Transplantation* 87, no. 10 (2009): 1429–35.

Index

advance directive. *See* living will

Alagille Syndrome, 141

alcohol, 16, 27, 28, 67, 92, 99, 106, 123

altruism, definition, 11, 18

altruism, examples: dolphins, 37; honeybees, 36; human infants, 37; termites, 37

altruism, theories of: altruism born of abundance, 89–90, 92; altruism born of suffering, 90–92; altruistic personality, 12; caring thinking, 74–78; code of conduct, 12; concern mechanism, 13; elevation, 160–62; empathy-altruism hypothesis, 14–15; genetics-based, 12, 36–38, 78, 92, 154; internalized personal values, 12–13; universal ethical principles, 12, 92; universal moral duty, 6, 37

anesthesia, 94, 109, 127, 128, 148

Batson, C. Daniel, 14

benefits, for the donor, 12, 13–15, 16, 38, 53, 109, 112, 153–54, 156, 160

bias, 33–34, 105, 111

blessed life. *See* bountiful life

blood donation, 1, 5, 6, 16, *17*, 22, 44–62 passim, 79–101 passim, 120, 138, 158, 160

bonding, donor-recipient, 23, 29, 42, 44, 48, 84, 147–48, 150

bountiful life, donor, 60, 64, 66, 90, 93, 102, 124, 138

brain, neuropsychology, 37–38, 78, 153–54

Brunt, Jan, 76

Buddhism, 34

California Living Donor Registry, 15, 168n11

cancer, 24, 49, 66, 67, 92–108 passim, 123, 149, 151

chain donation, vii, 25, 47–48, 60, 62, 80–81, 92

Church of Jesus Christ of Latter-day Saints, 93

clinical ethicist. *See* ethicist

coercion, 7, 34, 80, 107, 111

coincidences, donor-recipient, 28, 68

Comte, August, 12

concern, 11, 13–15, 18, 19–20, 53, 57, 60, 76

conflict of interest, 80, 105, 107

contentment, 47, 48, 60, 75, 89, 90, 107, 142

contraception, 134

"cooling off" period, 112–13, 145

cystic fibrosis, 20, 35, 41, 124, 151, 158

About the Authors

Katrina A. Bramstedt is a clinical ethicist specializing in organ donation and transplantation. She obtained her PhD in community medicine from Monash University Faculty of Medicine in Melbourne, Australia, and was an Ethics Fellow at the University of California Los Angeles. She counsels patients, families, and medical teams about complex medical ethics dilemmas and evaluates living donor candidates (www.AskTheEthicist.com). Her other book is *Finding Your Way: A Medical Ethics Handbook for Patients and Families.*

Rena Down is a professional playwright and screenwriter. She won an Emmy Award for directing "Voices" on PBS, and she has worked on several television series as story editor and producer and has written five movies for television. She has taught television writing at NYU's Tisch School of the Arts and Playwriting and Screenwriting at Mt. Holyoke College. Currently, she teaches screenwriting at The New School University in New York.